AF433916

Pregnancy Guide for First Time Moms

A Step-by-Step Guide to Healthy Pregnancy

Kimberly Ward

Table of Contents

Introduction 1

CHAPTER ONE

Are You Pregnant?...3

The Earliest Symptoms of Pregnancy 3
Pregnancy Tests...5

CHAPTER TWO

10 Common Pregnancy Questions 7

1. When is the right time for me to get pregnant?.......................7
2. What should I do if I am constipated during pregnancy?........8
3. Can I exercise while I am pregnant? 9
4. Can I drink alcohol? 9
5. Is sex safe during pregnancy? 10
6. Is it normal to have extra discharge during pregnancy?........11
7. Why am I always tired?..11
8. How to treat morning sickness? 11
9. How much weight should I gain?...12
10. How do I know if I am in labor? 12

CHAPTER THREE

Pregnancy Nutrition: What to Eat and What to Avoid 14

Key Nutrients 14
Foods to Eat During Pregnancy 16
Foods to Avoid During Pregnancy 18

CHAPTER FOUR

Healthy Pregnancy Recipes For Busy Moms...............................20

Breakfast...20
Cheesy Egg Wrap *20*

Oats with Banana and Strawberry 22

Simple Smoothie 23

Scrambled Eggs with Spinach 24

Buckwheat Dates Granola 25

Vegetables and Beans 27

Pasta and Artichoke Salad 27

Broccoli with Apple 28

Quinoa Casserole 29

Vegetarian Chili 31

Stuffed Bell Peppers 32

Meats and Seafood 33

Chicken Salad Sandwich 33

Mediterranean Baked Salmon 35

Balsamic Chicken and Beans 36

Instant Pot Beef Bourguignon 37

Beef Kebab and Rice 38

Tilapia with Veggies 39

Snacks and Dessert 41

Hummus 41

Tomato Bruschetta 42

Chocolate Mousse 43

Fruit and Nut Parfait 44

CHAPTER FIVE

First Trimester 46

Week 1 46

Week 2 47

Week 3 48

Week 4 49

Week 5 49

Week 6 50

Week 7 51

Week 8 52

Week 9 53

Week 10 54
Week 11 54
Week 12 56
Week 13 57

CHAPTER SIX

Second Trimester **58**

Week 14 58
Week 15 59
Week 16 60
Week 17 61
Week 18 61
Week 19 62
Week 20 63
Week 21 64
Week 22 65
Week 23 65
Week 24 66
Week 25 66
Week 26 67

CHAPTER SEVEN

Third Trimester **69**

Week 27 69
Week 28 70
Week 29 70
Week 30 71
Week 31 72
Week 32 73
Week 33 74
Week 34 75
Week 35 76
Week 36 76
Week 37 77

Week 38..77

Week 39..78

Week 40..79

CHAPTER EIGHT

Preparing for Labor and Delivery 80

Early Signs of Labor..80

Stages of Labor..81

C-section...83

Things to Have Prepared to Take to the Hospital.....................84

CHAPTER NINE

Postpartum: The First Days 86

Newborn Care..86

Taking Baby Home..87

Postpartum Recovery for Mom 89

Breastfeeding Basics 90

Burping Tips..92

Conclusion 95

Introduction

You're filled with joy—you have just found out you're expecting, and you can't wait to experience all the changes your body will go through as your baby grows inside of you. Then it hits you: you suddenly realize that you have no idea what to expect during your pregnancy.

It's okay. Although many of us experience different symptoms when we are pregnant, the same thing is going on inside our bodies. We are growing a tiny human and creating a new life right inside our wombs.

Whether you are already pregnant or thinking about getting pregnant, this book will walk you through the pregnancy so that you will take a proactive approach to your health and that of your baby. Chapter 1 explains the earliest symptoms of pregnancy and how to find out whether you are having a baby.

With all the changes occurring inside your body, it is only natural that you may feel a bit clueless about certain things. To put your mind to rest, Chapter 2 gives detailed answers to 10 common pregnancy questions.

What you eat during pregnancy has far-reaching consequences on your baby's development. Chapter 3 features the ideal pregnancy diet, the best foods to eat, and the foods to avoid. In Chapter 4, you will find 20 healthy and tasty pregnancy recipes for busy moms.

From Chapter 5 to Chapter 7, you will learn about what your body will go through each week of your pregnancy, as well as how your baby is changing. In Chapter 8, you will discover how to prepare for labor and delivery, including the signs of labor and what you need to take to the hospital. Finally, Chapter 9 prepares you for the first days after giving birth.

Being a first-time mom can engage an array of emotions, from feeling excited to overwhelmed and confused. By learning what to expect when pregnant, you will reduce some of those negative feelings to focus on the joy you will soon bring into your life.

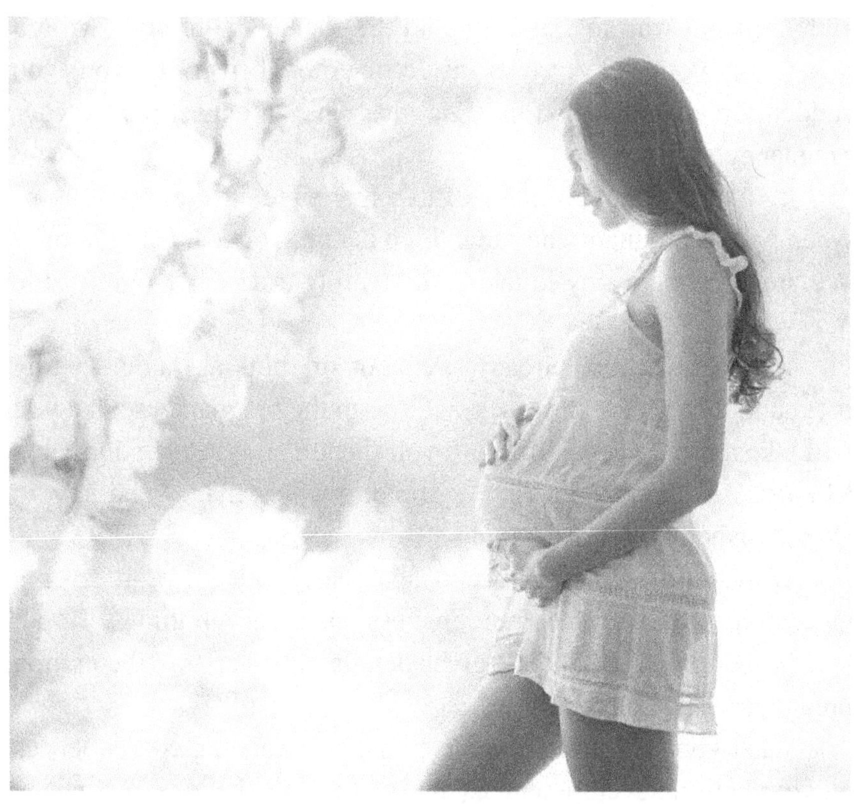

CHAPTER ONE

Are You Pregnant?

If you have been trying to conceive, then be on the lookout for signs of success. What seems insignificant may be an important clue. Just remember that the experience can differ among women.

The Earliest Symptoms of Pregnancy

1. Spotting

Once an egg is fertilized, it will try to attach itself along the wall of the uterus. This can trigger a bit of bleeding after one to two weeks. Check for spots of blood during this time. There might also be a white discharge throughout the pregnancy. This is a normal consequence of the rise in cell growth across the vagina's lining. If it comes with itching or a foul smell, consult your doctor to check whether there is an infection.

2. Cramping

The implantation bleeding can be accompanied by cramping. This can be hard to isolate as a pregnancy symptom since it feels just like menstrual cramps. Women might think that they are simply having the start of their period. The big difference is that the blood flow is light, and the cramps are not as painful.

3. Missed Period

Indeed, the regular monthly period will stop during your pregnancy. This is one of the biggest clues that send people in a hurry to get tested. Just remember that delayed or missed periods do not automatically point to conception. This could also be caused by hormonal imbalance, excessive stress, unhealthy weight loss, etc. Some forms of medication can also have this effect.

4. Breast Changes

You should pay attention to your breasts if you are trying to conceive. Pregnancy causes a sudden hormonal surge that generally results in sore and swollen breasts. They can feel tingly and tender. The nipples and their surrounding skin can get darker as well. The pain will subside after several weeks once your body adjusts to the hormonal changes.

5. Chronic Fatigue

It is also common for pregnant women to feel oddly fatigued soon after conception. This can be blamed on the rise of progesterone, a hormone produced by the ovaries. Contributing to this tiredness are other changes inside the body, such as reduced blood pressure and blood sugar, coupled with a rise in blood production. There is simply a higher demand for the body's depleted resources. Rest and nutrient-rich food are crucial.

6. Morning Sickness

Contrary to popular belief, not everyone will experience morning sickness during pregnancy. Some are lucky enough to go through the whole process without having this inconvenience. However, over half will have to wrestle with it, particularly in the first few months. Nausea can occur at any time, but it commonly happens in the morning, hence the name. Cravings and food aversions also tend to be stronger.

7. Frequent Urination

You may feel the need to pee more frequently than normal for a number of reasons. Sometimes it is due to diabetes or urinary tract infection. Others may experience it because of the consumption of diuretics. Pregnant women are likely to have this condition around 8 weeks after conceiving. It can be triggered by hormone changes and the growth of the uterus. The latter can put greater pressure on the bladder, forcing it to empty even at low volume.

8. Constipation

The rise in progesterone production has another undesirable consequence. Food will pass at a much slower rate through the intestines. This also means that solid waste will be harder to expel. Feeling constipated is not pleasant, so try to offset this by consuming more water and fiber-rich food. Exercise can also help in increasing blood circulation and boosting bowel movement.

9. Body Pain

A lot of women will experience recurring headaches while they are pregnant. Some also report feeling back pain. Take note of these physical discomforts. Observe when they started, when they usually happen, and what makes them go away.

Pregnancy Tests

While the symptoms above provide helpful clues, they are far from conclusive. Are you pregnant? Is it a certainty if you have cramps, constipation, or fatigue? Not necessarily. These could easily be caused by other conditions. The best way to find out whether you are having a baby is to take a pregnancy test. The following are some of the most commonly used modern approaches:

1. hCG Testing

The presence of human chorionic gonadotropin (hCG) in the blood or urine is a highly accurate pregnancy marker. It's a hormone that is made by the placenta right after implantation. Pregnancy strip tests are designed to detect it quickly. Note that hCG can also be produced by cancerous tumors. Those who are not expecting can use the strips as an initial test for cancer. These pregnancy kits are cheap and widely available.

2. EPF Testing

Although hCG testing is fast, simple, and accurate, it has flaws. The hormone will not be produced until the implantation of the fertilized egg has occurred, which could take several days. If the test is conducted before this, the result may be a false negative. If waiting is not an option for you, then a rosette inhibition assay for EPF or early pregnancy factor is a viable alternative. This method can be used within 48 hours of the egg's fertilization. It is rarely chosen because of the cost and complexity.

3. Obstetric Ultrasonography

Another method utilizes ultrasound technology to get a visual of the gestational sac and the embryo. A few weeks after gestation, it is already possible to view definitive forms in the mother's womb. Heartbeats can be seen within 6 to 7 weeks. For you and your partner, nothing is more fulfilling than seeing your unborn baby developing right before your eyes. This can be the final confirmation of your dream to have a new family member.

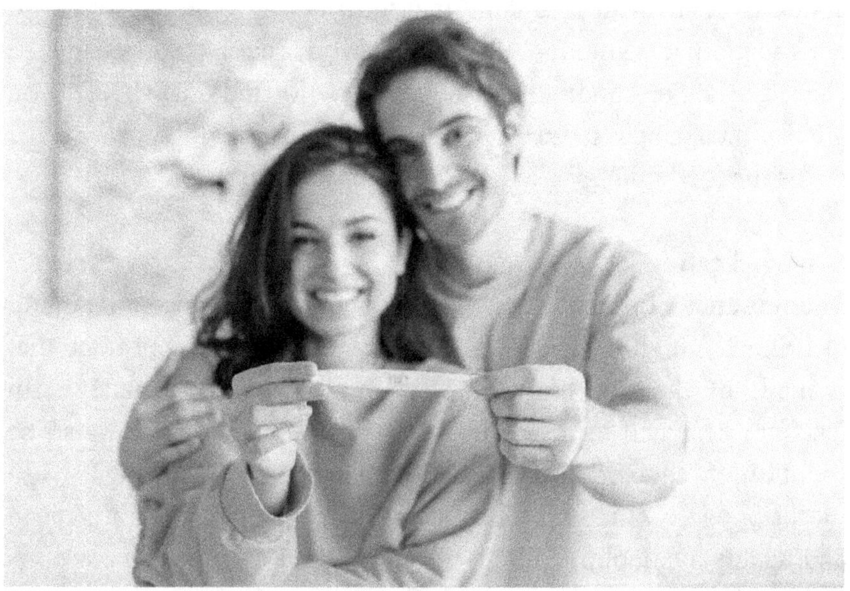

CHAPTER TWO

10 Common Pregnancy Questions

Being pregnant is a wonderful and unique experience for all would-be moms, but pregnancy also comes as an extremely challenging period for all women.

A whole host of changes occurs within your body, and it is only natural that the experience would make you feel a little weird, uncomfortable, and apprehensive about many things. You may often feel a bit clueless about certain things. To put your mind to rest, here are the answers to 10 common pregnancy questions.

1. When is the right time for me to get pregnant?

Your chances of getting pregnant are highest when you have sex in the period of 5 or 6 days leading up to the day of ovulation. The latter occurs typically during the middle of your menstrual cycle. If you have a regular cycle of 28 days, ovulation (when the eggs are released from the ovary) will occur about 14 days after your last period.

There is a reason why conceiving is most common during those 5 to 6 days (also called the "fertile window"). Once ovulation occurs, your eggs will survive for one to two days (in many women, only 12–24 hours), whereas the sperm released in your body has a normal survival rate of about one week.

So, having sex within that corridor means that when the egg is released, it will be ready to get fertilized by the spermatozoon. Having said that, one must also keep in mind that not all women enjoy regular menstrual cycles. With irregular cycles, it becomes much more difficult to determine the ovulation day. If this is the case with you, you should consider consulting a gynecologist.

However, if you enjoy an active sex life, the best practice is to have sex every 2 or 3 days. In this case, you won't have to worry too much about the other factors, and the pregnancy will occur on its own accord.

2. What should I do if I am constipated during pregnancy?

About half of all pregnant women suffer from the issue of constipation. So, if you have the same problem, there is no cause for alarm. Here is what you can do to prevent or ease constipation during pregnancy:

• Drink a lot of water and other fluids. Drink plenty of water or other light but healthy beverages throughout the day. Also, make sure to drink one or two glasses of fruit juice daily (grape and prune juice are the best options). Notice your urine color—pale yellow or clear urine is a sign of adequate hydration.

• Make sure to eat a lot of high-fiber foods. These include fresh fruits and veggies, beans, brown rice, and whole-grain bread and cereals.

• Drinking a cup of warm liquid the first thing in the morning, many suggest, eases constipation issues.

• During pregnancy, you will be prescribed a prenatal multivitamin. These vitamins are generally high in iron content, which can sometimes worsen the constipation problem in pregnant women. If you are suffering from constipation and not overly anemic, ask your doctor to prescribe a different vitamin or supplement.

• Keep up with some regular exercises. Brisk walk, swimming, yoga are some of the good options. But make sure not to overdo it.

3. Can I exercise while I am pregnant?

Not only you can, but ideally, you should follow some regular exercise routine during pregnancy. This will keep you mentally positive and healthy and help prevent or ease several health issues you may face during the pregnancy period.

But do not do something too strenuous. For example, you should never do weight exercises or anything else that may put too much stress on your abdomen. Go for lighter and cardiovascular routines. Good choices include stationery biking, swimming, light jogging, walking, and yoga.

However, if you are swimming, make sure not to dive into the pool. Also, you should gradually bring down the time of and the exertion caused by these physical activities during your second and third trimesters.

Though exercise is considered safe and even beneficial during pregnancy, if you have prior conditions such as hypertension, preeclampsia, heart disease, or preterm labor, it is best to keep your physical activities as limited as possible. Whatever the case, always consult your doctor before you start on any particular exercise routine during pregnancy.

4. Can I drink alcohol?

This is a tricky question. Some physicians advise complete abstinence during pregnancy, while others may say that occasional, light drinking is okay and is unlikely to harm your baby. You may also get differing opinions from already-moms. Some may say that they did indulge in occasional beers or other alcoholic beverages and their babies turned out fine. This question needs more scientific research, and there is no simple answer. However, the information from many different sources relates that an occasional sip of morning gin or a little champagne or wine during special occasions may be alright to most women.

If you can avoid alcohol altogether, nothing is better. On the other hand, if you are more or less habituated to drinking and enjoy it, then forcing complete abstinence on yourself may not be too good an idea since it may affect your mental health. Consult your doctor for suggestions if that is the case.

But remember, binge drinking or anything of that sort is a complete no-no since that can seriously affect your baby's health.

5. Is sex safe during pregnancy?

Yes, if you are enjoying a healthy pregnancy, having regular sex won't cause any harm whatsoever to your baby. Sometimes, you may feel that the baby moves a little after having an orgasm. But that is no cause for concern. The little creature is just reacting to the sudden increase in your heart rate.

There are occasions when you may want to be on your guard about having sex during pregnancy. For instance, expectant mothers who experience spotting or bleeding during early pregnancy are often advised by doctors not to have sex until they reach 14 weeks.

There are also a few special circumstances when you may need to stay away from sex completely during the entire period of your pregnancy. These circumstances are:

1. Vaginal infection during pregnancy
2. Regular heavy bleeding during pregnancy
3. A low-lying placenta
4. A history of cervical weakness

As with most other issues, it is best to consult your doctor first—just to be on the safe side!

6. Is it normal to have extra discharge during pregnancy?

Extra vaginal discharge, especially during the third trimester, is a normal side effect of pregnancy. There is no cause for alarm as long as your discharge is light and clear or of a pale yellowish color.

However, if you find that the discharge is somewhat thick or dense or has a strong odor, this may be a sign that you are suffering from yeast infection or Bacterial Vaginosis. In such cases, you should consult your doctor at the earliest.

7. Why am I always tired?

Fatigue or tiredness is one of the common symptoms during pregnancy. During early pregnancy, there is an increase in the progesterone hormone levels in your body. This hormone tends to relax the smooth muscles in your body, and it is therefore natural that you will feel somewhat sleepy or lacking in energy. Apart from the physical changes, the emotional changes you are passing through may also contribute to decreased energy and thus a feeling of tiredness.

Usually, the fatigue goes away during the second trimester, and it returns in the third. In short, unless you feel too out of sorts, fatigue or tiredness in itself is no cause for concern. Keep up with a healthy diet and moderate exercise, and you'll be alright.

8. How to treat morning sickness?

The best way to treat morning sickness during pregnancy is to alter your eating patterns. Keep a few crackers by your bedside (or make your other half prepare you some fresh toast first thing in the morning!) and eat some of them slowly before you leave the bed. This is found to help quell morning sickness.

Generally, following a diet high in carbs and protein helps combat nausea during pregnancy. Eat mashed potatoes, soda crackers, or brown bread and combine these carb-rich foods with protein such as cottage cheese with apple slices, hummus, whole pita, lean meat, etc., to avoid feeling exhausted throughout your day.

9. How much weight should I gain?

The right amount of weight gain is crucial during pregnancy. If you don't gain enough, the chances are that your baby will be of low birth weight. Gain too much, and you can run into complications like gestational diabetes. Typically, during the first 3 months of your pregnancy, you should gain 2–4 pounds and 1 pound a week for the rest of your pregnancy.

10. How do I know if I am in labor?

Although most babies are born between 37 and 42 weeks, there's no foolproof way to know when labor will begin. And this uncertainty often results in a lot of anxiety in expectant moms, especially first-time moms. Some common signs of labor include intense contractions at regular and frequent intervals (every 8 to 10 minutes) and lasting for 1–3 hours; losing of the mucus plug; water breaking; and bloody discharge (the "bloody show").

However, you may not experience all of these signs when you are in labor. If you have any doubt whatsoever, never take a chance and give a call to your doctor ASAP.

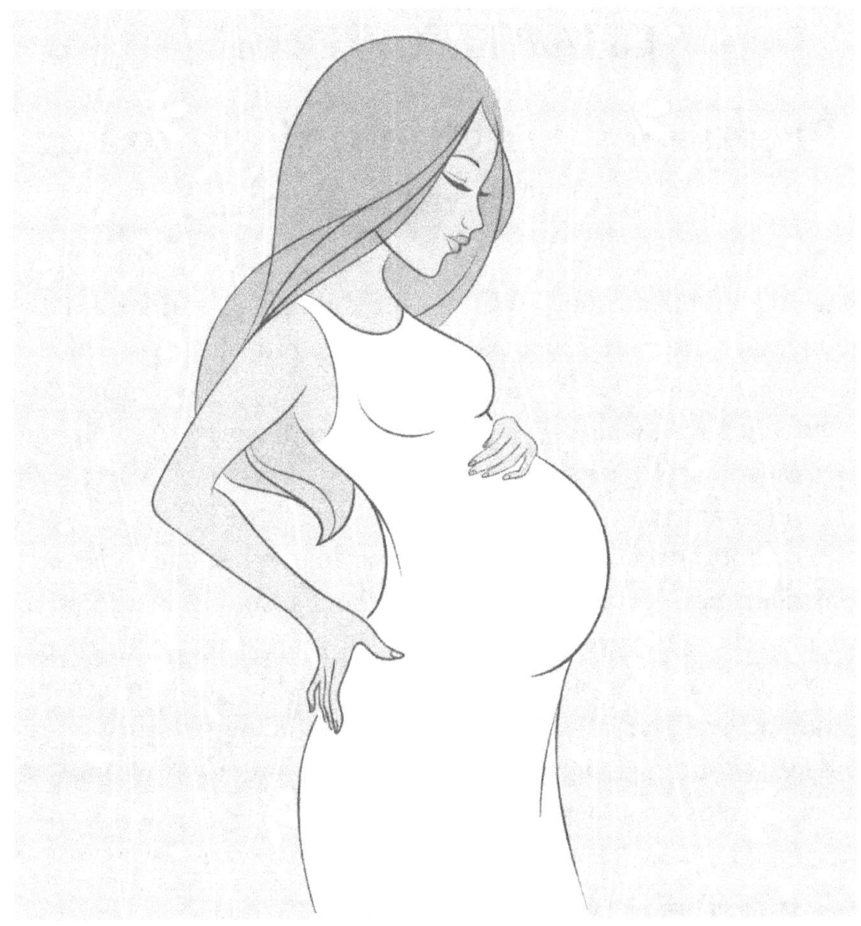

CHAPTER THREE

Pregnancy Nutrition: What to Eat and What to Avoid

It is no secret that eating a well-balanced diet is crucial for healthy living, more so during pregnancy. You are probably aware of the term "eating for two," which references how your meals are intertwined with your baby's nutrition. Indeed, what you eat during pregnancy has far-reaching consequences for your baby's growth and development.

For most women, the ideal pregnancy diet is one that feels great and nourishes your growing baby without resulting in excessive weight gain. However, creating a healthy pregnancy diet entails more than calorie restriction and often requires fine-tuning your eating habits. Currently, there's a lot of conflicting information on pregnancy diet and nutrition. This chapter provides a complete breakdown of what to eat and avoid.

Key Nutrients

Before we delve into the actual foods and drinks, it is crucial that you first understand the key nutrients and why they are essential. Generally, experts recommend that a mom-to-be eat a variety of healthy dishes and beverages, especially those rich in calcium, iron, folic acid, protein, and vitamins. Here's why these nutrients are vital.

Calcium

This mineral plays a crucial role in the growth and development of your baby's bone and tooth structures. Generally, a pregnant woman needs to consume at least 1000 milligrams of calcium daily, especially during the later stages of pregnancy. Dairy products such as milk, cheese, and yogurt are sufficiently rich in calcium. Leafy vegetables should also be a staple in your menu. Failure to consume sufficient amounts of calcium often leads to the mineral being extracted from the woman's bones which doesn't bode well for her body health.

Iron

During pregnancy, the blood volume in your body increases by almost 50 percent. To meet the extra demands of pregnancy, you need to consume twice the amount of iron you did before pregnancy. The mineral iron is required to make extra blood (hemoglobin) for you and the baby. Iron also helps the red blood cells to capture oxygen from the lungs for supply to your body and the baby's. A deficiency in iron during pregnancy can result in anemia, characterized by insufficient red blood cells. Anemia in pregnant women leads to fatigue and low immunity against illness.

Folic Acid

Folic acid, also known as folate, is a form of vitamin B9 that helps prevent severe congenital disabilities such as those of the brain and the spinal cord in your baby. Health experts recommend that pregnant women take at least 400 micrograms of folic acid before and during the entire length of pregnancy. The best source of folic acid lies in vitamin supplements, but fortified cereals and leafy vegetables can be just as good.

Proteins

The amino acids found in proteins act as the building blocks of your body and that of your developing baby. Besides cell growth, protein is essential for repairing damaged and worn-out cells, especially those in the brain and heart. It is critical that you make protein a key part of your diet, especially in the final 5 months of pregnancy.

Foods to Eat During Pregnancy

When it comes to nutrition, there's no such thing as the ultimate meal; the secret lies in consuming a wide variety of foods to ensure you never miss out on key nutrients. A healthy prenatal diet comprises the following groups: vegetables, fruits, dairy products, lean proteins, whole grains, and water.

1. Dairy Products

During pregnancy, you need to consume extra amounts of calcium, folic acid, and protein. Apart from being rich in calcium, dairy products also provide generous amounts of vitamin B, phosphorus, and zinc. Yogurt, in particular, is one of the best-known sources of calcium and also contains probiotic bacteria which support digestion while reducing the risk of vaginal infections. Therefore, it is recommended that moms-to-be take at least 3 servings of dairy products a day to get sufficient amounts of calcium, protein, and vitamin B.

2. Lean Meat

Chicken, beef, mutton, and pork are good sources of high-quality protein. Lean meat is also an excellent source of iron, choline, and a host of other vitamins, all of which are in high demand during pregnancy. Protein deficiency during pregnancy raises the risk of premature delivery and low baby weight. By consuming lean meat, you increase the amount of iron intake, which is crucial for blood production, especially during the third trimester of pregnancy.

3. Fruits

Fruits should be a key part of your diet, especially during the second and third trimesters. Fruits are ideal because they are rich in fiber, minerals, and vitamins. Oranges and grapefruits are particularly rich in vitamin C and folic acid. Berries, on the other hand, are packed with healthy carbs, water, and a generous amount of antioxidants.

Vitamin C, present in berries, plays a vital role in skin health and general body immunity. Additionally, fruits are a great snack due to their pleasant flavors and taste.

4. Leafy Vegetables

Leafy vegetables such as spinach, kale, and broccoli contain many nutrients that are hard to find in other foods. Calcium, iron, potassium, folic acid, vitamin C, vitamin A, vitamin K, and phosphorus are just examples of the many nutrients found in leafy vegetables. They are also rich in fiber which reduces the risk of constipation, a common issue among many pregnant women. Furthermore, greens contain antioxidants that aid digestion and boost immunity.

5. Eggs

Eggs make for a healthy meal mostly because they contain a little bit of almost every nutrient. A good-sized egg can provide up to 77 calories and a host of vitamins, fats not to forget high-quality proteins. However, the primary reason why eggs make this list is due to their high choline content. Choline plays a crucial role in your baby's brain development. Insufficient choline intake during the later stages of pregnancy can result in brain impairment and neural tube defects (spinal cord and brain defects).

6. Whole Grains and Legumes

Beans, peas, lentils, soybeans, peanuts, and chickpeas belong to a class of foods commonly known as legumes. Because legumes are rich in protein, iron, folate, and calcium, their intake can significantly reduce the risk of low birth weight and neural tube defects. Furthermore, legumes are generally rich in folate, which boosts immunity later in the baby's life. Whole grains, on the other hand, are ideal due to their high-fiber content.

7. Water

To facilitate the increase in blood volume, you need to be adequately hydrated throughout your pregnancy. Increasing your water intake helps to relieve constipation. Health experts recommend taking at least 1.5 liters of water a day; however, you can also get water from fruits and beverages such as tea and coffee. Failure to stay adequately hydrated leads to symptoms of headache, fatigue, and even anxiety.

Foods to Avoid During Pregnancy

1. Raw Meat

Uncooked and even undercooked beef, pork, and poultry can contain contaminants such as salmonella, toxoplasmosis, and a host of other bacteria which can be passed on to your baby. Some of these contaminants raise the risk of mental disability and impaired vision later in the baby's life. Raw shellfish, oysters, mussels, clams, and other undercooked seafood also pose serious health concerns to your baby's health. Raw eggs should also be avoided due to the high risk of passing salmonella to the baby.

2. Fish with High Mercury Content

Consuming foods with high mercury content can cause many complications to your unborn baby, such as poor brain development. As a result, pregnant women are advised to shun fish that contain high levels of methylmercury. This toxic chemical can easily pass through the placenta and affect your baby's development. Examples of such fish include marlin, king mackerel, swordfish, shark, and tilefish.

3. Unpasteurized Products

Consuming unpasteurized foods, especially dairy products, can lead to food poisoning. Unpasteurized milk, in particular, may contain a bacterium known as listeria. The bacteria is known to cause various complications such as miscarriage, preterm labor, and stillbirth. Deli meat and refrigerated food also pose similar risks. When you take milk and other dairy products, make sure it is pasteurized. Pasteurization entails applying heat to food products to kill bacteria and other disease-causing pathogens.

4. Alcohol

Prenatal consumption of alcohol usually interferes with the healthy development of the baby. Heavy alcohol use during pregnancy can lead to Fetal Alcohol Syndrome (FAS), a condition characterized by physical and mental impairment. Alcohol consumption is also discouraged for lactating mothers.

All in all, what you eat ultimately determines your health and your baby's wellbeing. It is essential for you to eat a variety of healthy foods and avoid harmful cravings. This will set you on the path towards a well-nourished pregnancy.

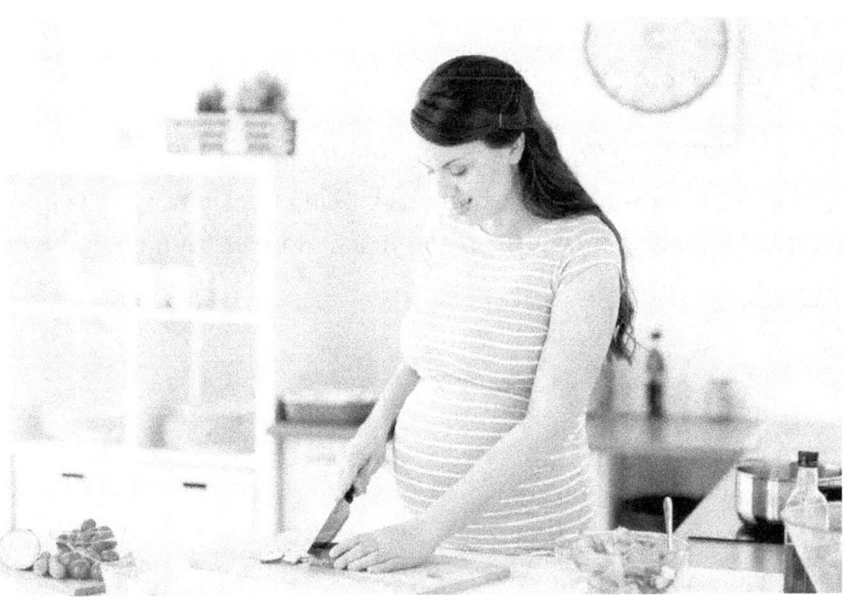

CHAPTER FOUR

Healthy Pregnancy Recipes For Busy Moms

Pregnancy is physically demanding. Women have to deal with a changing body, surging hormones, sudden cravings, and higher nutritional needs on top of their busy schedules. Clearly, self-care is essential throughout these 9 months. Make sure to eat healthy food to get enough energy, help the baby grow, reduce the risk of complications, and avoid runaway weight gain. Cooking at home is the best way to do this since you will have complete control over your meals. Don't worry if you don't have much time since you can always find easy options. Consider the following healthy and tasty pregnancy recipes:

Breakfast

Cheesy Egg Wrap

Eggs are breakfast staples. They are nutrient-dense, versatile, and easy to cook. However, you might be looking for a new way to enjoy these after simply frying them for years. How about a cheesy egg wrap?

Makes 2 servings
Ingredients:
4 eggs
1 cup tomatoes, diced
2 whole-wheat tortillas
1 cup baby spinach
1½ ounces cheddar cheese, shredded

1 onion, diced

2 teaspoons olive oil

Salt and pepper to taste

Directions:

1. Heat the olive oil in a pan.

2. Add the onions and spinach. Sauté until everything is a bit soft and wilted.

3. In a separate bowl, beat the eggs and pour them into the pan. Use salt and pepper to get your desired taste.

4. On a plate, put some of the cooked egg mixture in the middle of a tortilla. Sprinkle some tomatoes and cheese. Roll this up for a fresh Mexican-inspired treat.

5. You can get 2 to 4 servings depending on the amount of filling you place in each wrapper. This fast and easy breakfast can be eaten at home or on-the-go.

Nutritional Information (Per Serving)
Calories: 403
Fat: 21.8 g
Sat Fat: 7.9 g
Carbohydrates: 32.1 g
Fiber: 5.6 g
Sugar: 5.6 g
Protein: 22.2 g

Oats with Banana and Strawberry

Eating healthy means enjoying lots of fresh fruit. There's no cooking involved, just lots of luscious flavors.

Makes 5 servings

Ingredients:

1½ cups rolled oats

2 tablespoons walnuts, chopped

2 tablespoons dates, chopped

2 tablespoons shredded coconut

2 tablespoons chia seeds

1 banana, sliced

2 strawberries, sliced

1½ cups almond milk

1 tablespoon maple syrup

Directions:

1. Combine all dry ingredients in a bowl.

2. Place the fruit in a food processor and pulse until they liquefy.

3. Mix the fruit into the dry ingredients.

4. Add the almond milk and maple syrup and mix everything together.

5. Cover the bowl and refrigerate overnight.

6. Enjoy breakfast in the morning. If desired, add extra fruit or nuts.

Nutritional Information (Per Serving)
Calories: 355
Fat: 23.2 g
Sat Fat: 16.4 g
Carbohydrates: 35 g
Fiber: 7.5 g
Sugar: 11.1 g
Protein: 7.3 g
Sodium: 13 mg

Simple Smoothie

If you have a hard time eating breakfast, this smoothie recipe is a good option. Mix up the fruit selections if others are in season.

Makes 1 serving
Ingredients:
1 medium banana
1 cup strawberries
1 cup raspberries
½ cup plain yogurt
1 tablespoon honey
½ cup ice

Directions:
1. Mix all ingredients into a blender and combine on high until frothy.

Nutritional Information (Per Serving)
Calories: 366
Fat: 3.1 g
Sat Fat: 1.4 g
Carbohydrates: 78.6 g
Fiber: 14 g
Sugar: 52.8 g
Protein: 10.8 g
Sodium: 94 mg

Scrambled Eggs with Spinach

Boring scrambled eggs? These eggs will reawaken your taste buds.

Makes 2 servings

Ingredients:

4 eggs

1 tablespoon light cream

2 teaspoons olive oil, divided

1 garlic clove, minced

1 cup tomatoes, diced

1 cup baby spinach (fresh, not frozen)

1 tablespoon parmesan cheese, shredded

Salt and pepper to taste

Directions:

1. Whisk together the eggs, cream, salt, and pepper in a bowl.

2. Heat one teaspoon olive oil in a non-stick skillet over medium heat and sauté the garlic for 30 seconds.

3. Add the tomatoes and spinach and keep stirring until the spinach leaves are wilted.

4. Transfer to a bowl and cover with aluminum foil.

5. Heat one teaspoon olive oil in the same skillet. Add the eggs. Don't stir or "scramble."

6. When the eggs are set but still soft, top with the parmesan cheese and spinach.

Nutritional Information (Per Serving)

Calories: 219

Fat: 16.6 g

Sat Fat: 5.3 g

Carbohydrates: 5.5 g

Fiber: 1.4 g

Sugar: 3.1 g

Protein: 13.5 g

Buckwheat Dates Granola

Makes 12 servings

Ingredients:

2 cups oats

1 cup buckwheat groats

1 cup pumpkin seeds

1 cup sunflower seeds

1½ cups dates, pitted and chopped

1 cup apple puree

⅓ cup coconut oil

1 teaspoon fresh ginger, grated finely

¼ cup raw cacao powder

Directions:

1. Preheat the oven to 355 degrees F. Grease a large baking dish.

2. In a large bowl, add oats, buckwheat, and seeds, and mix well.

3. In a pan, mix together dates, apple puree, and coconut oil over medium-low heat. Simmer, stirring continuously for about 5 minutes until dates become soft.

4. Stir in ginger, immediately remove from heat, and set aside to cool slightly.

5. In a blender, add the date mixture and cacao powder and pulse until a smooth mixture forms.

6. Add the date mixture to the bowl with oat mixture, and stir to combine well.

7. Transfer the mixture to a baking dish. Bake for 15 minutes. Mix granola with a spatula.

8. Bake for 20–25 minutes until granola is crispy.

9. This granola can be preserved in an airtight container.

Nutritional Information (Per Serving)
Calories: 281
Fat: 13.3 g

Sat Fat: 5.5 g
Carbohydrates: 38.1 g
Fiber: 5.7 g
Sugar: 15.7 g
Protein: 7.6 g
Sodium: 5 mg

Vegetables and Beans

Pasta and Artichoke Salad

This salad has a zing that doesn't need any mayonnaise.

Makes 4 servings

Ingredients:

8 ounces spiral pasta

¼ cup frozen peas, thawed

1 tablespoon lemon juice

3 teaspoons olive oil

1 can chopped artichoke hearts

8 ounces mozzarella cheese, diced

⅓ cup roasted red bell pepper, chopped

Directions:

1. Cook the pasta according to directions. When done, add the peas.

2. Mix the lemon juice and olive oil together in a bowl. Stir in the remaining ingredients.

3. Mix in the pasta and peas.

4. Serve warm or at room temperature.

Nutritional Information (Per Serving)

Calories: 435

Fat: 14.5 g

Sat Fat: 6.7 g

Carbohydrates: 51.4 g

Fiber: 4 g

Sugar: 2.9 g

Protein: 25.1 g

Sodium: 442 mg

Broccoli with Apple

Makes 4 servings

Ingredients:

1 tablespoon olive oil

2 garlic cloves, minced

2 cups small broccoli florets

½ cup red onion, chopped

¼ cup celery stalk, chopped

¼ cup low-sodium vegetable broth

2 apples, cored and sliced

Directions:

1. In a large skillet, heat the olive oil over medium-high heat.
2. Add garlic and sauté for about 1 minute.
3. Add broccoli and stir fry for about 4–5 minutes.
4. Add celery and onion and stir fry for about 4–5 minutes.
5. Stir in the vegetable broth and cook for about 2–3 minutes.
6. Add apple slices and cook for about 2–3 minutes.
7. Serve hot.

Nutritional Information (Per Serving)

Calories: 105

Fat: 3.7 g

Sat Fat: 0.5 g

Carbohydrates: 18.6 g

Fiber: 3.9 g

Sugar: 12.7 g

Protein: 1.1 g

Sodium: 56 mg

Quinoa Casserole

Enjoy healthy quinoa and lentils in this casserole.

Makes 8 servings

Ingredients:

2½ cups quinoa, cooked according to package instructions

2 cups lentils, cooked according to package instructions

1 onion, diced

3 garlic cloves, minced

1 tablespoon olive oil

10 ounces fresh spinach

2 cups tomatoes, diced

2 eggs

½ cup plain Greek yogurt

6 ounces feta cheese, crumbled

3 teaspoons dill

Salt and pepper to taste

Directions:

1. Heat the olive oil in a skillet and sauté the onions and garlic for a few minutes.

2. Stir in the spinach. Cover and cook for 5 minutes.

3. When the spinach is wilted, remove it from heat.

4. Preheat the oven to 375 degrees F.

5. Mix together the cooked lentils and quinoa, the spinach, and tomatoes.

6. In another bowl, whisk the eggs and add the yogurt and feta. Season with dill, salt, and pepper.

7. Stir the quinoa/lentil mixture into the egg mixture and mix thoroughly.

8. Transfer to a casserole dish and bake for 40 minutes.

Nutritional Information (Per Serving)

Calories: 480
Fat: 11.3 g
Sat Fat: 4.2 g
Carbohydrates: 69 g
Fiber: 20 g
Sugar: 4.2 g
Protein: 26.9 g

Vegetarian Chili

Makes 8 servings

Ingredients:

2 cups onion, diced

1 cup celery, diced

1 cup bell pepper, diced

2 cloves garlic, minced

2 tablespoons olive oil

1 jalapeño pepper, diced

4 cups crushed tomatoes, no salt added

2 cups canned pinto beans, drained and rinsed, no salt added

2 cups water

2 teaspoons cumin

1 teaspoon chipotle pepper

1 tablespoon balsamic vinegar

1 tablespoon oregano

Salt and pepper to taste

Directions:

1. Add onion, celery, bell pepper, and garlic in 2 tablespoons of olive oil in a stockpot over medium heat. Cook until onions are translucent.

2. Add the rest of the ingredients. Cover and simmer for 1–2 hours, occasionally stirring.

3. If chili becomes too thick, thin it with water, adding small increments of water at a time.

Nutritional Information (Per Serving)
Calories: 123
Fat: 4.3 g
Sat Fat: 0.6 g
Carbohydrates: 18.4 g
Fiber: 5.2 g
Sugar: 4.9 g

Protein: 4.7 g

Stuffed Bell Peppers

Makes 4 servings

Ingredients:

½ pound shiitake mushrooms

1 cup celery stalk

2 garlic cloves, peeled

½ cup walnuts, chopped

2 tablespoons olive oil

Pinch of salt

Freshly ground black pepper to taste

4 small red bell peppers, halved and seeded

Directions:

1. Preheat oven to 400 degrees F. Grease a baking sheet.

2. Remove stem and seeds from bell peppers.

3. In a food processor, add mushrooms, celery, garlic, walnuts, oil, salt, and pepper and pulse until finely chopped.

4. Stuff bell peppers with mushroom mixture.

5. Arrange bell peppers onto the prepared baking sheet.

6. Bake for about 20–25 minutes.

Nutritional Information (Per Serving)
Calories: 232
Fat: 16.7 g
Sat Fat: 1.6 g
Carbohydrates: 19.6 g
Fiber: 4.3 g
Sugar: 8.6 g
Protein: 6.1 g
Sodium: 199 mg

Meats and Seafood

Chicken Salad Sandwich

This is a great recipe to make use of leftover rotisserie chicken, although you can always cook things fresh as well. If you prefer seafood, you can also substitute low-mercury fish or crab sticks as the protein source.

Makes 4 servings

Ingredients:
8 bread slices
1½ cups cooked chicken, chopped
½ cup celery, chopped
1 onion, diced
½ cup mayonnaise
½ cup cucumber slices
½ cup carrots, shredded
4 lettuce leaves
Salt and pepper to taste

Directions:
1. Combine the cooked chicken, carrots, celery, onion, and mayonnaise in a bowl. Use salad dressing instead of mayo if you prefer.

2. Add a pinch of salt and pepper to adjust the taste. You may also use other herbs and spices.

3. Put lettuce and cucumber slices on a piece of bread. Scoop some of the chicken mix into these and top off with another slice of bread.

4. Take this to the office for a filling lunch. This should make 4 servings in total so you can share with family or co-workers.

Nutritional Information (Per Serving)
Calories: 328

Fat: 22.3 g
Sat Fat: 3.6 g
Carbohydrates: 14 g
Fiber: 1.7 g
Sugar: 3.1 g
Protein: 17.2 g

Mediterranean Baked Salmon

This dish combines the goodness of salmon with green salad ingredients. What could be better?

Makes 4 servings

Ingredients:

4 salmon fillets

2 tablespoons olive oil

2 tomatoes, diced

2½ tablespoons feta cheese, crumbled

3 tablespoons red onion, diced

½ tablespoon chopped basil

1 tablespoon lemon juice

Directions:

1. Preheat the oven to 350 degrees F.

2. Brush the salmon with olive oil and place it in a baking dish.

3. Top the fillets with the remaining ingredients and bake for 20 minutes. The salmon should be flaky.

Nutritional Information (Per Serving)

Calories: 321

Fat: 18.8 g

Sat Fat: 3.5 g

Carbohydrates: 3.4 g

Fiber: 0.9 g

Sugar: 2.3 g

Protein: 36.1 g

Sodium: 152 mg

Balsamic Chicken and Beans

Makes 4 servings

Ingredients:

4 skinless, boneless chicken breasts

¼ cup balsamic vinegar

2 garlic cloves, minced

2 shallots, sliced

3 tablespoons extra-virgin olive oil

1 pound fresh green beans, trimmed

1 tablespoon red pepper flakes

Directions:

1. Combine 2 tablespoons of olive oil with the balsamic vinegar, garlic, and shallots. Pour it over the chicken breasts and refrigerate overnight.

2. The next day, preheat the oven to 375 degrees F.

3. Take the chicken out of the marinade and arrange it in a shallow baking pan. Discard the rest of the marinade.

3. Bake in the oven for 40 minutes.

4. While the chicken is cooking, bring a large pot of water to a boil. Place the green beans in the water and allow them to cook for 5 minutes, and then drain.

5. Heat 1 tablespoon of olive oil in the pot and return the green beans after rinsing them. Toss with red pepper flakes.

Nutritional Information (Per Serving)

Calories: 433

Fat: 17.4 g

Sat Fat: 3.3 g

Carbohydrates: 12.9 g

Fiber: 4.6 g

Sugar: 3.1 g

Protein: 56.1 g

Sodium: 140 mg

Instant Pot Beef Bourguignon

Makes 4 servings

Ingredients:

1 pound beef stew meat

4 bacon slices

2 garlic cloves, minced

2 medium onions, chopped

4 medium carrots, chopped

2 tablespoons parsley

2 tablespoons thyme

½ cup beef stock

1 cup red wine

2 large potatoes, cubed

1 tablespoon honey

1 tablespoon olive oil

Directions:

1. Place the oil in the Instant Pot and select SAUTÉ. Add beef and cook for 3–4 minutes or until browned. Set the beef aside.

2. Add bacon and onion, and sauté until onion is translucent.

3. Add beef and the rest of the ingredients and close the lid.

4. Cook at high pressure for 30 minutes.

5. When the cooking is complete, do a natural pressure release.

6. Serve warm.

Nutritional Information (Per Serving)

Calories: 541

Fat: 17.9 g

Sat Fat: 5.2 g

Carbohydrates: 47.8 g

Fiber: 7.7 g

Sugar: 12.3 g

Protein: 36.9 g

Sodium: 662 mg

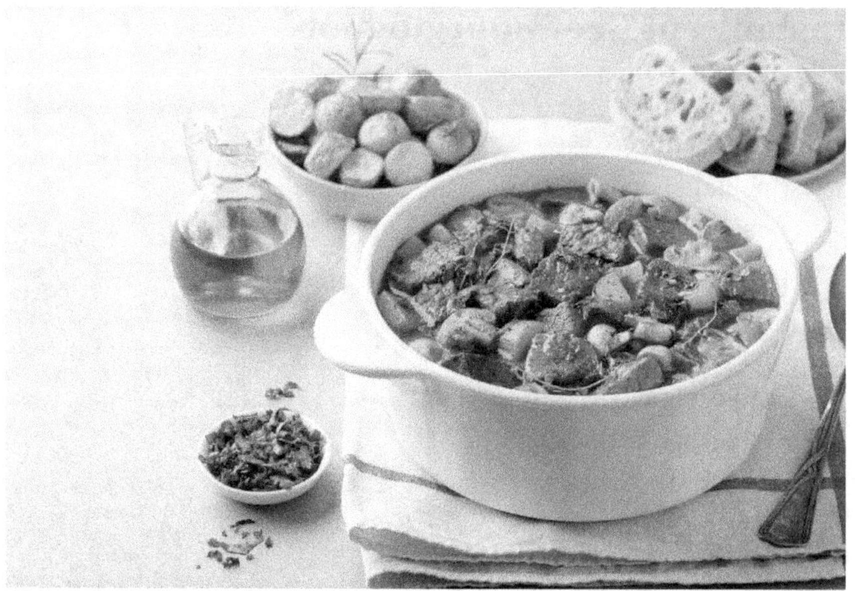

Beef Kebab and Rice

Makes 4 servings

Ingredients:

½ pound lean beef

12 cherry tomatoes

12 button mushrooms

1 red onion

2 tablespoons soy sauce

2 tablespoons lemon juice

1 tablespoon olive oil

1 teaspoon cumin powder

4 cups brown rice, cooked

Directions:

1. Create the marinade by mixing the soy sauce, lemon juice, and cumin.

2. Cut the beef into one-inch cubes and soak them in the mixture overnight. If you can't wait until the next day, give it at least 3 hours to absorb the flavors. You can also substitute lean cuts of pork for the beef if you want to.

3. Once you are ready to cook, set up the grill and let it reach high heat. Place the ingredients in the metal skewers by alternating the meat with the cherry tomatoes, onion, and mushroom. You can also use pineapple chunks and bell pepper slices.

4. Grill these kebabs until tender. Be sure to turn them in every few minutes for even cooking.

5. Put one kebab per plate with a cup of brown rice.

Nutritional Information (Per Serving)
Calories: 328
Fat: 8.4 g
Sat Fat: 1.9 g
Carbohydrates: 39.7 g
Fiber: 2.9 g
Sugar: 3.6 g
Protein: 23.5 g
Sodium: 501 mg

Tilapia with Veggies

Makes 2 servings
Ingredients:
2 (3-ounce) tilapia fillets
1 cup zucchini, sliced
1 cup summer squash, sliced
1 cup tomato, sliced
1 cup red bell pepper, seeded and sliced
1 cup red onion, sliced
2 tablespoons fresh rosemary, minced
Pinch of salt

Freshly ground black pepper to taste
3 teaspoons olive oil

Directions:
1. Preheat the oven to 350 degrees F. Grease a large baking dish.
2. Place all ingredients except for oil in a large bowl and toss to coat.
3. Transfer the mixture into the prepared baking dish.
4. Bake for about 20–25 minutes.
5. Transfer the mixture to a serving plate.
6. Drizzle with oil and serve.

Nutritional Information (Per Serving)
Calories: 220
Fat: 8.9 g
Sat Fat: 1.7 g
Carbohydrates: 19.9 g
Fiber: 5.8 g
Sugar: 11 g
Protein: 19.3 g
Sodium: 152 mg

Snacks and Dessert

Hummus

Hummus is a versatile dip that you can pair with sliced vegetables, pita bread, crackers, or anything you like. It is a vegan-friendly snack with a decent amount of protein and good fats.

Makes 8 servings

Ingredients:
1 can garbanzo beans (15½ ounces)
2 tablespoons tahini
4 tablespoons lemon juice
2 tablespoons olive oil
2 cloves garlic
Salt and pepper to taste

Directions:
1. Start by chopping the garlic cloves in a blender. Add garbanzo beans, lemon juice, tahini, and some liquid from the can to get your preferred creamy consistency. Blend until smooth.

2. Put more liquid if it seems too thick. Add salt according to your taste.

3. Once you are satisfied, transfer the hummus to a bowl and sprinkle pepper on top. You can also pour the olive oil in a circular fashion.

4. Try dipping veggie slices in it and enjoy. Some people use hummus as a substitute for salad dressings and pasta sauces. It can also add creaminess to soups and mashed potatoes.

Nutritional Information (Per Serving)
Calories: 109
Fat: 6.1 g
Sat Fat: 0.9 g
Carbohydrates: 11.4 g

Fiber: 2.4 g
Sugar: 0.2 g
Protein: 3 g

Tomato Bruschetta

Yield: 6 servings

Ingredients:

½ whole-grain baguette, cut into 6 (½-inch-thick) slices on the diagonal

3 tomatoes, chopped

½ cup fennel, chopped

2 garlic cloves, minced

1 tablespoon fresh parsley, chopped

1 tablespoon fresh basil, chopped

2 teaspoons balsamic vinegar

1 teaspoon olive oil

Freshly ground black pepper to taste

Directions:

1. Preheat the oven to broil. Arrange a rack in the top portion of the oven.

2. Arrange bread slices on a baking sheet in a single layer.

3. Broil for about 2 minutes per side.

4. Meanwhile, in a bowl, add remaining ingredients and toss to coat.

5. Divide the tomato mixture evenly and place it on each slice of toasted bread. Serve immediately.

Nutritional Information (Per Serving)
Calories: 94.5
Fat: 1.5 g
Sat Fat: 0.1 g
Carbohydrates: 18 g

Fiber: 2.5 g
Sugar: 1.0 g
Protein: 3.7 g
Sodium: 176 mg

Chocolate Mousse

As an occasional treat, dark chocolate works well for pregnant women with a craving. It's not too sweet, and it even has antioxidants. Make it even better by pairing it with protein-rich Greek yogurt.

Makes 6 servings

Ingredients:
2 cups Greek yogurt
2 tablespoons honey
1 cup low-fat milk
1½ cups dark chocolate
pinch of salt

Directions:
1. Use a food processor to chop the chocolate fast.
2. In a boiler, mix the milk, honey, and salt over medium heat. Be careful to prevent it from boiling.
3. Add the chocolate and stir until everything has melted, then remove from heat.
4. Drain excess liquid from the yogurt and place it in a mixing bowl. Pour the chocolate into this bowl and stir to get an even mixture.
5. Divide the contents into 6 containers and chill for a few hours before serving.

Nutritional Information (Per Serving)
Calories: 299

Fat: 12.7 g
Sat Fat: 7.8 g
Carbohydrates: 30.1 g
Fiber: 3.8 g
Sugar: 24.5 g
Protein: 16.5 g
Sodium: 93 mg

Fruit and Nut Parfait

Makes 4 servings
Ingredients:
1 cup melon
1 banana
1 cup mixed berries
¼ cup raisins
½ cup walnuts
2 cups fat-free vanilla yogurt

Directions:
1. Cut the melon into chunks about the same size as your berries and slice the banana. Mix in a large bowl with the raisins and walnuts.
2. Top with the yogurt and blend to combine.
3. Chill for 30 minutes before serving.

Nutritional Information (Per Serving)
Calories: 253
Fat: 10.5 g
Sat Fat: 1.1 g
Carbohydrates: 33.7 g
Fiber: 3.7 g
Sugar: 24.9 g
Protein: 10.4 g
Sodium: 104 mg

As you can see, eating healthy doesn't have to mean settling for bland food. You can make nutritious and delicious meals in your kitchen. Just make sure to pick quality ingredients whenever possible. Feel free to modify the recipes based on what you have in your pantry or what your taste buds dictate. The more you make them, the easier they will be as you get used to the process. If you have special considerations such as allergy and illness, consult your doctor or dietician for recommendations.

CHAPTER FIVE

First Trimester

The amazing thing about becoming pregnant is that you are considered pregnant on the first day of your last monthly cycle, even though the egg has yet to be fertilized. This is how a doctor will calculate your due date and determine how far along you are. A pregnancy is divided into 3 trimesters, totaling about 40 weeks. Your first trimester is from weeks 1 through 13.

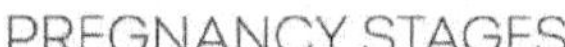

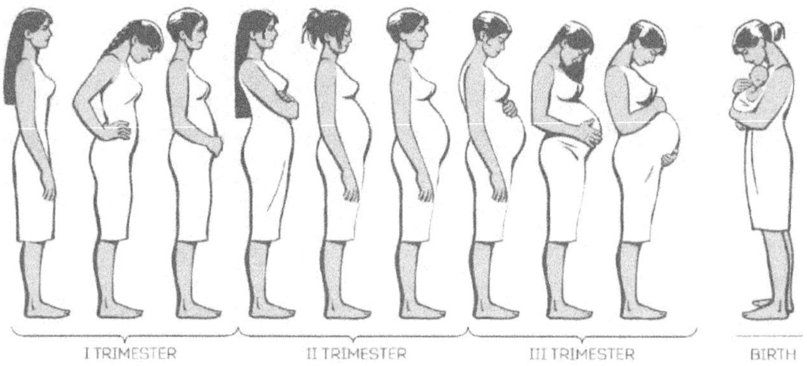

Week 1

This is the week of your cycle, and the first week doctors will count when determining how far along you are and your due date. However, you are not technically pregnant at this point. Conception usually takes place 14 days after the first day of your period. When your doctor calculates your estimated due date, they will ask for the first day of your last period and add 9 months to that day, plus 7 more days.

If you are planning on getting pregnant, this is the time for you to make sure you begin to practice healthy habits, such as eating more fruits and vegetables, drinking plenty of water, taking vitamins containing folic acid, and ensuring that your vaccinations are up to date.

You should make sure you are not smoking or drinking alcohol, that you cut back on your caffeine consumption, and avoid all hazardous materials. You should also talk to your doctor to ensure you are not taking prescription medications that could harm your baby. However, you should never stop taking medications without your doctor's approval. Your doctor will be able to weigh the benefits of the medication against the chances of it affecting your baby and decide whether you should continue taking the medication or if your medication should be changed.

Week 2

At 2 weeks pregnant, you are still not technically pregnant yet. The lining of your uterus is beginning to thicken as your body prepares to release an egg. This is the time of the month you are most likely to get pregnant, but it is important to know that the average woman only has about a 25 percent chance of getting pregnant at this time. This percentage reduces with age, as a 30-year-old woman only has about a 15 percent chance of becoming pregnant at this time, and a woman approaching 40 only has about a 10 percent chance. Often it is actually less, depending on the health of the person.

When the uterine lining thickens, it is getting ready to provide nourishment and protection for the baby it anticipates. Your body is about to release an egg, ready to be fertilized, in a process known as ovulation. After the egg is released, there is a window of 12-24 hours to become fertilized. After this time, your next chance at becoming pregnant won't occur until the following month.

If fertilization does occur, it creates what is referred to as a zygote, which is simply a single cell that begins to travel down your

Fallopian tube to the uterus. While the zygote is moving into the uterus, it will begin dividing itself into more cells, which ends up looking very much like a small raspberry. This process happens extremely quickly. There are 2 groups of cells at this point, the inner cells that will form the embryo and the outer cells that will be used to protect and nourish the embryo.

Right now, your baby is growing very quickly, forming tiny systems, such as the digestive system.

Week 3

Congratulations, you are now officially pregnant! Although you are probably completely unaware of the miracle taking place inside your body, your egg has been fertilized, and in a few short months, you will have a brand new baby!

During the third week, the egg is called a blastocyst, and has divided into hundreds of cells, all from that single-cell zygote! This group of cells will implant itself into your uterine wall during this week, which will provide the embryo with the nutrients it needs, and remove waste, as well.

Eventually, this implantation site will become what we know as the placenta and will provide the nutrition your baby needs while you are pregnant. It is important for you to focus on your health during this time and ensure you and your baby are getting the proper nutrients.

You can experience early pregnancy symptoms, but they often get overlooked because they resemble PMS symptoms. Some of the early pregnancy symptoms include breast tenderness, mood swings, fatigue, and aching in the lower abdomen. It is no wonder most women do not realize they are pregnant at this point, as they are already expecting their period.

It is during this time when there can be some spotting, often referred to as implantation bleeding. However, not every woman experiences this, and even those that have experienced it in past pregnancies may not experience it in future ones.

Week 4

Surprise! You missed your period. This is when most women find out they are pregnant. However, because of implantation bleeding, some women do not realize they have missed their period until the following month. This is why your doctor will ask you if there were any noticeable differences in your last period. This allows them to know, even if you did not, that you did not actually have a period but experience implantation bleeding instead.

If you have an extremely light period about a week to a few days before your period is supposed to begin, you can take a pregnancy test at week 4 to determine if you are pregnant. Most store-bought home pregnancy tests are just as accurate as the test you would take at the doctor's office and are often as accurate as a blood test.

At this point in your pregnancy, you may notice that your breasts are tender, and you have to urinate more frequently. You may also feel fatigued and suffer from mood swings. Most women do not notice any weight gain at this point, but they may feel as if they are slightly bloated.

You now have an embryo, and the baby's brain, spinal cord, and organs are starting to form, even though the embryo is only .04 inches in size.

Week 5

By this time, most pregnancies have been confirmed by a pregnancy test. The embryo's nervous system is beginning to develop, the head is becoming distinct, the heart actually begins to beat, and the bones are beginning to develop. The baby is now .06 inches long, or the size of an apple seed.

You may begin to experience morning sickness at this point. Your breasts will still be tender, and you will still need to urinate often. You may experience fatigue and suffer from headaches caused by hormonal changes taking place in your body. It is important to know that you may not experience any of these symptoms at all. The symptoms of pregnancy vary from one person to the next, and they can even vary from one pregnancy to the next, so not having symptoms is not something that should cause you to worry.

Starting this week, you will need to eat an additional 300 calories per day, focusing on healthy foods, such as fruits and vegetables. You should avoid some foods, such as soft cheeses, unpasteurized milk, undercooked or raw meat, deli meat, hot dogs, anything containing raw eggs, and all raw fish and seafood.

Week 6

It is during this week you may find your symptoms becoming worse. This is because the baby is growing so rapidly and can be as big as .16 inches. You may suffer from symptoms such as morning sickness or nausea, food cravings may begin, and you may start to find certain foods do not appeal to you the same way they used to. You may also find you are extremely fatigued, and your breasts will still be tender, but they may also begin to tingle and ache as well.

You can now recognize your baby's head in an ultrasound, as well as see the tiny limb-buds that have begun to form. The eyes, nose, ears, and mouth are also beginning to form during this week, as are many organs, such as the lungs, liver, and thyroid gland.

Now is the time for you to become aware of the signs of a miscarriage, including bleeding, cramping or sharp pains in the stomach, and passing blood clots. Many women have a bit of spotting throughout their pregnancy, so there is no reason to think that every spot of blood means you may be having a miscarriage. However, you need to contact your doctor if you have any of the signs of a miscarriage so they can ensure the baby is okay and give you peace of mind.

This period of your pregnancy is critical when it comes to the development of your baby's organs. You should ensure you stay away from nicotine, caffeine, hair treatments such as hair coloring that might cause you to inhale chemicals, as well as other beauty treatments that use chemicals, and avoid changing the kitty litter.

If you do not have a prenatal visit set up with your doctor yet, now is the time to make the appointment.

Week 7

When you are 7 weeks pregnant, you are still in the second month of your pregnancy. Your baby has increased to the size of a small marble and currently weighs .03 ounces. You may find you are still suffering from morning sickness or nausea, and you may be salivating excessively, have vaginal discharge, and your waistline will begin to expand slightly. However, your pregnancy will not be physically visible at this point. If you suffer from morning sickness, you may also find that you have lost a few pounds, but this is perfectly normal and will not affect your baby's development. Many women lose weight during their pregnancies, but as long as your doctor monitors the baby's development, there is no reason for this to cause concern.

On the other hand, some women find they are beginning to gain weight at this point in the pregnancy. It is important to monitor your weight gain to ensure you do not put on too many pounds. A woman of average weight before she becomes pregnant should only gain about 25 pounds throughout pregnancy. One underweight should gain about 30 pounds, and a woman who was overweight before becoming pregnant should gain about 15 pounds through the entire pregnancy.

During this week, your mucus plug will develop over the opening of the cervical canal, sealing the uterus off to protect the baby. This plug will be lost when your body prepares for labor.

At this point, your baby's heart has completely formed. The baby's eyelids are forming folds, the tongue is beginning to form, the pituitary gland begins forming in the brain, and the cerebral cortex can now be seen.

Week 8

During the eighth week, your baby is about the same size of a pumpkin seed. You will most likely have your first prenatal visit. Your uterus is growing and is now about the same size of an orange, so you may notice that your jeans are beginning to fit a bit tighter around the waist.

You may notice you have acne caused by the increase of hormones in your body. Your breasts may become tender and swollen, you may still suffer from morning sickness and nausea, as well as extreme fatigue, and you could develop a pooch in your tummy.

During a first pregnancy, most women don't show at this point; however, in later pregnancies, you may begin to start showing early on because your muscles and ligaments have already been stretched in previous pregnancies.

Lots of things are going on with your baby. The bud of the legs begins to divide into 3 separate sections—one for the thigh, one for the calf, and one for the foot. The arm-buds start to divide into separate sections for the arms, as well.

The baby's arms and legs will begin to move, teeth begin to form under the gums, and the gonads also begin to form.

During your first prenatal visit, you will be weighed and asked to give a urine sample. Your blood will be taken, the nurse will check your blood pressure, and you will be asked to change into a gown.

Your doctor will do a cervical exam, which is much like a pap smear. Though this can be very uncomfortable, it does not put your baby or your pregnancy in any danger. Your doctor will prescribe prenatal vitamins as a supplement for your nutrition and that of your baby. However, this does not mean that you can eat poorly. Instead, continue to focus on getting the proper nutrition for both you and your baby.

At the end of the exam, you will be asked to make a follow-up appointment, and it is vital to the health of you and your baby that you keep these appointments. Make sure that before your doctor leaves the examination room, you ask any questions you may have. It is a good idea to write these questions down ahead of time and take them with you, as it is easy to forget what you wanted to ask once you've walked into the examination room.

Week 9

During this week, your baby has grown to about the size of a paper clip and weighs about 1 ounce. Hair follicles will begin to form this week, the upper lip will develop, the neck will become distinct, and movements can be seen on an ultrasound.

Your breasts become fuller and more sensitive. You may notice a small amount of weight gain, and you might also begin suffering from heartburn. You may find you are dealing with some cravings and that some of the foods you once loved are no longer desirable to you. It is at this point that you may become emotional, crying for no reason and suffering from mood swings.

During the first trimester, many women go through changes in their sexual desires, some wanting to participate in sexual activities more often, some less, and some not wanting much to do with it at all. This is entirely normal, but if you are concerned about the changes, be sure to talk to your doctor.

Week 10

Congratulations! You are now ¼ of the way through your pregnancy. Your baby will be very busy growing this week, with the brain producing around a quarter of a million neurons every minute! Your baby weighs about as much as a quarter. Most of the little body parts are present, too, but they are tiny.

During this week, your baby's ears will be completely formed. Males will start producing testosterone, and the ovaries in females will begin to descend. The baby's fingers and toes will be separate instead of webbed. The skeletal system continues to develop, the roof of the mouth forms, taste buds begin to form, and the diaphragm starts to develop.

Make sure you drink at least 64 ounces of water every day. The amount of blood in your body is going to increase by about 50 percent, which may cause your veins to become more noticeable, especially on your breasts and stomach, and often on your legs as well. You may also find your complexion is a bit blotchy, you may still be dealing with mood swings, you will begin to notice a bit more weight gain and the softening of your gums.

Week 11

Once you have reached the 11-week mark, the embryo is now called a fetus because the majority of critical development is now complete. Your baby will grow very rapidly, and by the end of the week, the baby will be about 2 inches long. For your body to accommodate this rapid growth, the blood vessels in the placenta increase in number and size, providing the baby with more nutrients.

You have been pregnant for 80 days and have about 200 more days to go until you finally hold your baby in your arms.

During this week, the baby's eyelids will fuse closed, remaining this way until you are about 24 weeks pregnant. The genitals have moved to the outside of the baby's body, the baby develops hair follicles on the skin, and teeth are still forming.

The baby's head is about half the size of the entire baby because the brain has developed. The ears will begin moving up from the sides of the neck to the sides of the head.

By this week, you should have gained about 5 pounds, although some women gain 10 or more during the first trimester because they stop worrying about trying to keep the weight off. However, gaining a large amount of weight does come with consequences. When you gain extra weight, it does not benefit the baby but turns to fat instead, which will be very difficult for you to get rid of after giving birth. Gaining too much weight can pose a health risk to you and your baby. Carrying around excessive weight can put you at risk for gestational diabetes and stress your organs as well as your blood vessels.

You should have your second prenatal visit. You will likely have an ultrasound and hear your baby's heartbeat for the first time. Expect your doctor to track your blood pressure because having high blood pressure during pregnancy can lead to preeclampsia, a severe health issue. Your doctor will also take a urine sample every month to check for infection and protein in the blood, which may be a sign of high blood pressure. They will also check for sugar in the urine, which can mean that you have gestational diabetes. Your doctor will measure the size of your uterus by pushing on the abdomen to locate the top of the uterus. This will allow the doctor to know the baby's size and ensure it matches the expected due date.

Your breasts will be very tender and feel very full. You may also notice that the skin color around your nipples is darkening due to the increased supply of blood, which causes your veins to become more visible and is perfectly natural. It is a good idea to ensure you find a very good support bra at this time. Consider looking for a maternity bra.

You may also notice you are suffering from dizziness or nausea as well.

Week 12

You have almost completed your first trimester, and this is when people may begin to tell you that you are glowing. This pregnancy glow is because of the increase of blood supply in your body and can cause you to look plumper and make your skin look smoother.

The great news is that your chances of miscarriage have dropped dramatically. Most of the time, if there is going to be a miscarriage, it will occur before this point. This is why most people wait until they are about 12 weeks pregnant before announcing their pregnancies.

At this point, your baby has grown to about 2.5 inches. This may not seem very big, but in the past 3 weeks, your baby has doubled in size.

Your baby's gallbladder is beginning to secrete bile, and the lungs have finished forming. The liver is now making blood cells and takes up about 10 percent of the baby's weight. The baby urinates for the first time, and the intestines are now in the abdomen. Your baby's muscles have developed, and he or she will spontaneously twitch.

Because of the extra oil secretion, you may find your acne has increased, but this can be relieved using an over-the-counter acne treatment. During this week, the baby will shift upwards and forward, which means the baby will no longer be pressing down on your bladder, and you will have to go to the bathroom less often.

You may also find you are suffering from morning sickness less often, you have more energy, but you may also suffer from headaches or lightheadedness.

Since the physical symptoms are easing, this is a good time for you to start focusing on light exercise. Exercise is great for both you and your baby. However, you want to make sure that you do not overdo it.

Week 13

You have made it to the last week of the first trimester! You might begin to notice you have developed a baby bump. Your morning sickness, as well as the mood swings, will be getting better if they have not disappeared altogether.

Your baby is about 3 inches long and can move arms and legs. The baby might also bring a thumb to the mouth, although the baby is not able to suck on it.

The baby will also start to develop fingernails, as well as fingerprints. The vocal cords start forming this week, too, and the eyes will move closer together on the face. The ribs will become visible, and the organs will finish developing.

You may also find that you are suffering from anxiety, though less often than before, due to the lower risk of miscarriage. You may feel some discomfort in your abdomen because of the stretching of the ligaments that hold your uterus, but this is completely normal. If you are still suffering from fatigue, it is perfectly normal, and simply your body is getting used to being pregnant.

CHAPTER SIX

Second Trimester

Your second trimester lasts from week 14 to the end of week 26. Most women find the second trimester easier than the first one.

Week 14

This is the first week of your second trimester, and your baby is now either male or female. This is the week when you should start to feel better and have more energy, but you may still have to deal with a bit of constipation. You may find that you have gained a few pounds. Your hormones should become more balanced, which will help reduce the amount of nausea or morning sickness you are dealing with and the amount of exhaustion.

Your baby is around 4 inches long. Your baby will begin to grow fine hair over the entire body, called lanugo, which is shed before the baby is born. The vocal cords have finished developing, and the thyroid gland will start to produce hormones. The baby will also start inhaling and exhaling, and the hands will become more functional. The baby now receives all nutrients from the placenta, which has taken the production of hormones over from the ovaries.

If you find that constipation has become a problem, you should ensure you are getting enough water in your diet, as well as healthy, fiber-rich fruits and veggies. You may also find that the veins in your breasts are becoming more visible, the nipple area may increase in diameter, your breasts may become larger due to the new milk ducts forming, and they may feel heavier and sore. This may also cause the nipple to become more sensitive as well.

Many women find that by the end of this week until the end of the pregnancy, they produce more body heat, which causes them to feel warmer. You may also find you often have to deal with headaches. These are known as hunger headaches caused by a drop in blood sugar. To avoid these, make sure you are eating healthy snacks regularly.

Week 15

By the time you reach the 15th week of pregnancy, your baby will weigh around 1.7 ounces. You may have a "baby bump" at this point, as well as headaches or nosebleeds on a regular basis. This is completely normal and will pass in time.

Many women look forward to looking visibly pregnant at this point, but if you have not started to show yet, don't worry. It will come with time. You may, however, find you are having a hard time zipping or buttoning your pants, but that you are not yet ready to start wearing maternity clothes. If this happens, you can use what is known as the rubber band trick, where you will slip a rubber band through the buttonhole in your pants and then place both ends of the rubber band around the button.

Your baby will be able to move the arms and bend them at the elbows and wrists. It is also possible for your baby to make a fist. By now, your baby's legs have become longer than the arms, and eyebrows, as well as the hair on the scalp, will appear. The skeletal system continues to develop.

There are many changes going on with your body as well. You may find you have abdominal pain as your uterus grows, your breasts may begin leaking, and you may discover hair and skin changes. To ease the abdominal pain, apply heat, avoid sudden movements, and make sure you stand up and sit down slowly.

A yellow liquid called colostrum may begin to leak from your breasts. This is the first milk your baby will drink, containing many antibodies that will help protect him or her from disease. If the leaking becomes bothersome or your clothes are getting stained, you can purchase nursing pads to place inside of your bra. During this time, you need to make sure you keep your breasts clean, washing them in warm water to avoid crust from forming around the nipple from the colostrum.

If you suffer from nosebleeds, it is often because of the increased blood flow in your body, but this can be avoided by keeping the air moist with a humidifier.

Many women also find their hair has begun to grow faster and thicker, while others find it becomes easily dirty, thins, and becomes drier. Hormones may cause these changes in your hair, and if they are bothersome, the best thing you can do is look for a shampoo that focuses on the issue bothering you, be oily hair or dry.

Week 16

You may feel what many call butterflies in your stomach, but which is your baby moving. This usually starts between this week and the 22nd week of pregnancy, so do not worry if you do not feel anything right away.

This is a good week to discuss the different genetic tests available with your doctor.

Your baby is a bit over 4 inches long and weighs about 3 ounces. Your baby can now open the mouth, as well as move lips, and even swallow. This is when your baby may begin sucking his or her thumb. The baby will begin to make a variety of facial expressions, and the heart rate will increase to 157 beats per minute. If the baby is a female, millions of little eggs will begin to form inside the ovaries.

You may find that your nose is stuffed up, your gums may begin to bleed, your feet may swell, and you may experience abdominal pain due to the stretching of the ligaments.

Week 17

During this week, your baby's hearing will begin to develop. The baby will start to hear not only what is going on inside of your body but also what is going on outside of your body. This is a great time to start talking to your baby, playing music, and singing to him or her.

You may begin feeling more energetic due to the placenta producing all of the hormones your body previously was in charge of producing. Your baby is just under 5 inches long and weighs about 3.5 ounces at this point. Your baby's heart will be pumping about 6 gallons of blood each day!

Your baby will begin breathing amniotic fluid. However, the baby's oxygen supply is provided through the placenta. The circulatory system is working, and the baby is quickly developing reflexes.

You should have gained anywhere between 5 and 10 pounds, your appetite is increasing, and your lower abdomen is beginning to swell. You may also be completely over morning sickness and any food aversions you previously experienced.

Week 18

During this week, your baby's growth rate will begin to slow down, but the baby's reflexes are still quickly developing. Your baby is between 5 and 6 inches long and weighs about 5 ¼ ounces. Even though your baby is very small, your uterus has grown to about the size of a cantaloupe.

The baby will begin to produce feces, which will be stored in the colon. The baby's skeleton can clearly be seen on an ultrasound. The ears are noticeable on the sides of the head, and the pads on the fingertips and toes are beginning to form. The baby's bones are also starting to harden, so it is important to ensure you are getting enough calcium.

Your baby can also hear very well at this point because the bones in the inner ear and the nerve endings have developed, which means the baby can hear your heartbeat and even your blood as it moves through the umbilical cord.

You may feel your baby moving, and you may even see your stomach jerking when your baby has hiccups.

Week 19

At 19 weeks pregnant, you have almost made it to the halfway point. Your baby is about 6 inches long and weighs 7 ounces, about the same weight as an orange! Now your baby is able to purposefully move muscles, bringing his or her hand to the mouth and sucking the thumb. However, there are still some involuntary muscle movements. If you have not felt your baby move yet, do not worry, as many women do not feel their baby move until they are about 26 weeks pregnant.

You should have another prenatal checkup around this time in which the doctor will weigh you, check your blood pressure, ask for a urine sample, check your uterus, and check your baby's heartbeat. You should have gained about 10 to 13 pounds.

Your doctor may also talk to you about a condition called anemia. There are 2 different types of anemia often seen in pregnancy, one being the type caused by the lack of red blood cells. The second one, iron deficiency anemia, is caused by the lack of iron found in the body, which means that you need more iron. It is important for you to answer your doctor's questions honestly, especially when they ask about what you eat because poor eating habits can lead to anemia. Other reasons include having several pregnancies in a short amount of time, carrying multiples, and even having morning sickness.

Your doctor can give you a blood test to determine if you are suffering from anemia, but common symptoms include pale skin, a feeling of breathlessness, fainting, fatigue, and the feeling that your heart is pounding. Treating anemia is very simple—your doctor will have you begin taking an iron supplement. You can also improve the amount of iron in your body by eating whole grains, beans, leafy greens, spinach, and dried fruit.

During this week, your baby is developing millions of nerves that connect to the brain, the legs will begin to grow in proportion to the rest of the body, and the skin is transparent. Vernix, a thin, white, creamy coating that protects the baby's skin from scratches as well as from becoming chapped in the liquid environment, will begin to form around the baby.

You may find you have blotchy skin on your face, the skin on your belly may become dry and itchy, you may develop a rash on areas where your skin has stretched, and you may begin to see stretch marks. There are no miracle lotions to prevent stretch marks. However, keeping the skin moist will help prevent itching and irritation and soften the skin. The best way to avoid stretch marks is to eat healthily and drink lots of water throughout your pregnancy.

You may also notice abdominal pain, dizziness, leg cramps, heartburn, swelling in the feet, as well as backaches.

It is usually at this point in the pregnancy that men and women begin to worry that sex may cause harm to the baby. The fact is that sex will not harm your baby at all, and as long as you have a healthy, normal pregnancy, sex is safe.

Week 20

This week, you may notice your baby has started to move around a lot more. The baby weighs about 9 ounces and is about 6 ½ inches long. Your baby can hear, and you will be able to feel him or her jump when startled by a loud noise.

Hair continues to grow on the head, so do the eyebrows. The skin begins to form layers, and the nails on the fingers and toes start to grow. If the baby is a female, the uterus will begin to develop this week.

You may feel as if your body no longer belongs to you. This is something many women experience, but do not worry, as in a few short weeks, it will be all yours again.

The line from your belly button to your pubic bone may begin to darken, but this will fade after the baby is born. You may begin sweating more due to changes in your thyroid gland and may notice the need to urinate more often. Other issues that may be bothersome for you are shortness of breath, indigestion, and heartburn, as well as vaginal discharge, a change in complexion, and a change in the appearance of your belly button.

Week 21

You have finally passed the halfway point in your pregnancy! Your baby now weighs about 10 ½ ounces and is about 7 inches long. The baby's growth rate will slow, but the baby's organ system will continue to develop.

Most of the baby's nourishment is still coming from the placenta, but at this point, his or her intestines will begin to develop small amounts of sugar and water, which are absorbed back into the amniotic fluid. Your baby will swallow the fluid, which will pass through the digestive system, but it will go no further than the large intestine.

Your baby's skin and organs will develop this week. The heart grows stronger, and the baby will begin to produce brown fat, which will help maintain body temperature. The baby will also begin to develop buds for permanent teeth.

You may find you suffer from constipation caused by the hormone progesterone. This makes it take longer for things to pass through your digestive system, making the stools harder than usual. During this time, you are at a higher risk for urinary tract infections. You may notice your feet and ankles begin to swell, and you may suffer from hemorrhoids. Often women report their gums have become sensitive, too.

Week 22

From this point to the end of your pregnancy, you will gain weight at a steady rate. Your baby is now about 12 ounces in weight and about 8 inches long.

Playing your favorite music during this time will help soothe your baby after birth. When a baby hears the same sounds that he or she heard while in the womb, the baby will become comforted. So this is a great time to turn on Classical music.

During this week, the baby's eyelids and eyebrows become further developed, the fingernails are entirely formed, and taste buds begin to form. If the baby is a boy, the testes have begun to descend into the scrotum; if the baby is a girl, she has already developed about 7 million eggs in her ovaries.

You may find your body has begun to practice for delivery. You may have painless contractions, called Braxton Hicks. Not all women have Braxton Hicks, but having them is nothing to worry about. On the other hand, if you have painful contractions or more than 4 per hour, you need to contact your doctor.

Week 23

At 23 weeks, your baby is now about 8 inches long and weighs about a pound. Your baby will begin to move the fingers and toes, and arms and legs, which you may feel. Often, if you look down at your stomach, you may see the movements.

From this point forward, your baby will gain about 6 ounces per week. The baby will also develop more distinct lips and eyes this week. The bones located inside the middle ear will begin to harden, and pigments will be deposited into the baby's skin.

Even though your baby's head is still out of proportion to the body, starting this week, the body and the head will start to become more proportional.

Some of the symptoms you may be experiencing are trouble sleeping, heartburn, frequent urination, itchy skin, leg cramps (which may be relieved by eating bananas), anxiety, mood swings, and vaginal discharge.

Week 24

By the end of this week, your baby can weigh as much as 1.5 pounds and be about 8.5 inches long! The baby can use all of the senses and is developing blood vessels in the lungs. Your baby is also developing eyelashes and will begin producing white blood cells. The baby's inner ear has completely developed.

At this point, your breasts are swelling as they prepare to make milk, and the area around your nipples may become larger and darker. You may find you are suffering from leg cramps, heartburn, lower back pain, constipation, and forgetfulness, as well as having a difficult time sleeping.

You should have another prenatal visit, where your doctor will ask for a glucose test and a urine sample, check your weight, blood pressure, the baby's heart rate, and the size of your uterus.

Week 25

At 25 weeks pregnant, your baby will weigh about 1.5 pounds and be about 9 inches long. You only have 2 more weeks until you begin your third trimester! You will probably feel your baby moving around a lot as well.

Your baby will continue to gain weight, and the skin will begin to look more like your own instead of the translucent skin the baby has had up until now. The spinal cord is starting to form, the taste buds continue to form, and the hands have become fully developed. The nostrils are also beginning to open up.

Your uterus has grown to about the size of a soccer ball. You may experience hemorrhoids, which can be helped with over-the-counter medication, but you should talk to your doctor if you are concerned. You may also suffer from dizziness, heartburn, forgetfulness, constipation, increased sweating, and very vivid dreams.

Week 26

By now, your baby has grown to about 9.2 inches in length and is about 2 pounds. It is important to make sure you are getting enough sleep and getting plenty of healthy fruits and vegetables in your diet and lots of water. You have to remember that your baby depends on you for everything, which means you have to take care of yourself.

Your baby will begin to look more like when he or she is born. The baby will spend the next 14 weeks putting on fat and preparing for delivery. The baby's eyes will unseal, and the baby will begin blinking. The baby will also begin mimicking breathing, although there is no actual air entering the lungs. The baby will also respond to touch.

After this week, you will gain about 1 pound per week, and you may begin to suffer from side pain caused by the stretching of your abdomen.

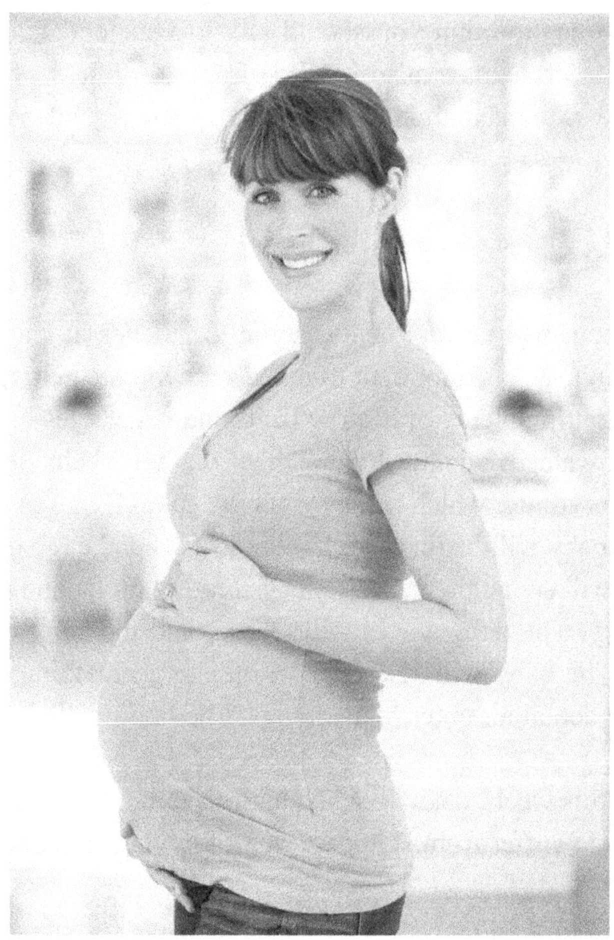

CHAPTER SEVEN

Third Trimester

Congratulations! You have made it to the third trimester and have only a few more weeks to go. The great news is that if your baby is born this week or later, he or she would have at least a 90 percent chance of survival and would look much like a baby born at 40 weeks, albeit smaller and thinner.

There is still a lot of development that must occur during the next 13 weeks. Often babies born during this gestational period are unable to breathe on their own, which means they have to stay in the hospital much longer than one born at full term.

Week 27

At this point in your pregnancy, your baby weighs a little over 2 pounds and is just under 10 inches long. The brain will begin to grow rapidly, the nerves that connect to the ears are fully developed, and the baby is breathing amniotic fluid. The baby starts to recognize your voice, as well as that of your partner.

You should have gained between 16 and 22 pounds. You may find you are having a hard time with balance, but you need to take your time and be careful, to ensure you do not fall. If you have developed stretch marks, they will become more visible during this week.

Although it may seem like delivery is far off, now is the time to start making plans. You may decide to take some childbirth classes, especially if you are a first-time mom.

Week 28

Your baby can weigh anywhere from 2 to 3 pounds and is about 10 inches in length, from the top of the head to the buttocks, or about 15 inches from head to toe. During this week, your baby will grow about ½ of an inch in length.

Your baby will begin to dream, often moving as he or she is dreaming, which means less sleep for you. The baby is now up to about 3 percent body fat, and the muscles are becoming stronger throughout the body. Even though the lungs are very small, they are capable of breathing in the event of premature delivery. However, the baby would still require medical treatment.

You should have another prenatal visit with your doctor, who will ask for a blood sample, check your weight, blood pressure, and the size of your uterus, as well as the baby's heart rate.

The average weight gain at this point in pregnancy is anywhere from 17 to 24 pounds. You may suffer from leg cramps, known as restless leg syndrome. Bananas are a great way to treat this, as potassium helps relieve the cramps.

You may also suffer from shortness of breath, clumsiness, abdominal pain, heartburn, the need to urinate frequently, and Braxton Hicks contractions.

Week 29

There are only 12 more weeks to go, and you will be holding your bundle of joy in your arms. You should expect to put on about 10 more pounds before delivering the baby. It is important to keep your size in mind as you are going about your daily routines—there will be no more slipping through small spaces, and you might find you bump into things more often. If you need help from your partner, you should not be afraid to ask.

Your baby has grown to about 10.5 inches from the top of the head to the buttocks and weighs about 2 pounds and 12 ounces.

Your baby will be moving more often, and some of the kicks can be breathtaking. If you are afraid there has been a reduction in movement, you can do what is called a fetal kick count, where you count the number of times you feel the baby move in an hour. You should feel the baby move at least 10 times. If you do not, you should contact your doctor.

By now, your baby has learned how to breathe, so if born prematurely, the baby would most likely be able to breathe on his or her own. Your baby can now turn the head from left to right and is becoming more sensitive to the sounds in and out of the womb. Fat layers continue to form on the baby's body, and the head is now proportionate to the rest of the body. The baby's eyes can move, and the bones are fully developed but not completely hardened.

Ensure you are getting enough iron, phosphorous, and calcium in your diet so that your baby has all the nutrients needed.

You may find you are short of breath and have itchy skin, as well as indigestion, muscle cramps, and hemorrhoids. You may also experience pain in the pelvic area due to the uterus growing. You will usually feel this pain on the inside of the thighs and around the groin area, often occurring with exercise, lifting of the legs, and even getting out of bed. It can also happen when you laugh, cough, or sneeze.

Week 30

Take advantage of your alone time with your partner because, after the birth, chances are it will be a while before you have this opportunity again. You may also spend some time planning and preparing for the birth of your baby. This is also when most new mothers become restless as they wait for their baby to arrive.

Your baby is now about 11 inches in length from the top of the head to the buttocks and weighs about 3 pounds. From this week on, the baby will gain an average of ½ a pound per week.

The baby's head is growing larger, the thin hair on the baby's body is beginning to fall out, although there will still be some patches on the back and the shoulders. The baby spends most of the time with the eyes open, looking around.

The baby will begin to mimic your breathing and will often inhale amniotic fluid, which can cause hiccups, but this is nothing to be concerned about.

Most mothers complain about suffering from constipation. To avoid this, make sure you get enough exercise and eat foods containing a lot of fiber. These foods include vegetables, fruits, and grains. You should also make sure you drink plenty of water. If constipation does not resolve itself, talk to your doctor about taking a stool softener.

During this week, you will develop more stretch marks, your body will swell, and you will most likely suffer from heartburn.

Week 31

With only 10 more weeks to go, your baby weighs about 3 pounds, 8 ounces, and is about 11 inches long from the top of the head to buttocks. After this week, your baby will not grow as quickly as in previous weeks, but the baby will still gain about 2 more pounds before birth.

Your baby's lungs and the digestive tract are almost fully developed. The baby can see the inside of the womb, and the eyebrows and eyelashes have completely come in as well.

You should have a prenatal visit during this week. Talk to your doctor about Braxton Hicks contractions, as well as any other concerns you may have. As your pregnancy progresses and you grow closer to your due date, these contractions may intensify, causing you to worry about premature labor. However, these are just practice contractions as your body prepares to go into labor.

During the visit, the doctor will take a urine sample, weigh you, measure your blood pressure, check the size of your uterus, and check the baby's heart rate.

You should have put on about 19 pounds in total up to this point. Your body is going through further changes besides the weight gain, which may include the development of varicose veins, leaky breasts, and a vaginal discharge that may get heavier as the pregnancy progresses.

Week 32

At 32 weeks pregnant, you only have 9 more weeks left in your pregnancy, and it may feel as if your body is changing every single day. Your baby should weigh about 4 pounds by now and is around a foot in length from the top of the head to the buttocks.

Since your baby is growing and taking up more space in the uterus, there will be less room to move around, which means that you may not feel movement as frequently as you previously did, and when you do, the kicks may not be as strong. If you are concerned that your baby is not moving around enough, you can practice kick counting, looking for no less than 10 kicks in a two-hour period. If you find that the baby is not moving at least 10 times within 2 hours, you should immediately contact your doctor.

Your baby will continue to develop layers of fat underneath the skin. The arms and legs should be fully developed and proportionate to the baby's size. The hair on the baby's head will continue to grow, and the thin hairs that once covered the baby's body have almost completely fallen out.

You may still be suffering from heartburn, indigestion, or breathlessness. You may find you are retaining fluid throughout your entire body. If you see spots or small flashing lights while you are resting, experience sudden swelling in the face, suffer from stomach pain, nausea, or vomiting, you must contact your doctor.

These are all signs of preeclampsia, which is a severe health issue that could lead to your death or the death of your baby.

It is important to discuss your birth plan as delivery comes closer. It is a good idea to have your birth plan written down so that your partner, as well as your nurses, know what you will need. This is also a good time to start making a list of the items you want to take with you to the hospital.

Week 33

Up until this point, you have gained anywhere from 22 to 28 pounds. During the next several weeks, expect a further weight gain of about a pound a week as your baby more than doubles in size before you give birth.

At this point, your baby is about 12 inches long and weighs about 4.5 pounds. The baby may have a full head of hair and develop normal sleeping patterns. However, many times, this means the baby is sleeping during the day and active at night, which will make it harder for you to sleep.

The baby can hear sounds, can see the inside of the womb and has feelings. The lungs are almost completely developed, and they will function properly outside of the womb now. The baby continues to develop fat, and the skin turns from red to pink during this week.

You may feel as if your belly will pop at any moment. It may look as if it might, but don't worry, as it will all return to normal after you deliver your baby. You may find you are exhausted, suffer from Braxton Hicks, as well as pelvic pain caused by the pressure your baby is putting on your pelvic area.

It is common for women to have wildly vivid and strange dreams at this point of their pregnancy and a decreased interest in sex.

This is a good time for you to start to think about how you will deal with the pain during delivery, and you might find it helpful to speak with your doctor about pain relief options.

Week 34

At this point, it may seem as if it will be an eternity before you can hold your baby in your arms, but the truth is you only have a few weeks left! The baby has now positioned with the legs curled up to the chest in the fetal position because space is quite limited.

Though the baby has not yet turned into the birthing position, you still have plenty of time to prepare for his or her arrival. If your baby is born at any time after this week, chances of survival are very high. However, the baby would probably have to be on oxygen, as well as in an incubator, but rest assured—the most dangerous time for premature labor has passed.

Your baby weighs about 5 pounds and is almost 13 inches long from the top of the head to the buttocks. The baby's skeleton will harden, although the skull will remain pliable to allow passage through the birth canal. The baby's skin will reduce in redness, and the developing fat underneath it will fill out the wrinkles. The fingernails have grown to the tips of the fingers by this point, and the baby is beginning to develop immunities that will allow him or her to fight mild infections.

You may begin to feel anxious about the upcoming delivery and the responsibility of taking care of your new baby. Your body may also suffer from aches and pains, and you will continue to gain about 1 pound per week.

During the last weeks of your pregnancy, you should try to rest as much as possible. Do not drink caffeine to stay awake because it can negatively affect the baby. Take frequent naps when needed. You may also have to deal with pelvic pain, sore ribs, and Braxton Hicks.

Week 35

You should have gained anywhere from 24 pounds to 29 pounds. Your baby weighs about 5.5 pounds and is around 12 inches in length. Ninety-nine percent of babies born at this week of pregnancy survive.

During this week, your baby will store fat all over the body, the lungs are almost fully developed, and the baby will be in the head-down position, ready for delivery.

You may not be sleeping well, suffer from mood swings, and become more irritable. Most of this is the result of physical discomfort. You may also suffer from hemorrhoids and constipation.

Week 36

Only 5 more weeks to go—that is, if your baby does not come early or late. The reality is that only 5 percent of all babies are born on their expected due date

You may begin feeling a bit overwhelmed at this point in your pregnancy. You may find that you are beginning to experience nesting, starting to obsessively clean and prepare your home for your baby. Some women find they constantly wash and fold the baby's clothes as they wait for delivery. You may also find your belly is becoming very itchy. This can be relieved by applying a lot of lotion.

Your baby weighs about 6 pounds and is about 13 inches from the crown of the head to the buttocks. The baby should have already dropped into the birth position, which can cause extra pressure on your lungs, as well as your stomach. It can also cause a slight tingling in the pelvic area and the legs. You will probably have increased backaches, as well as constipation and heartburn.

You should have a prenatal examination this week for your doctor to weigh you, check your blood pressure, collect a urine sample, check the size of your uterus, and perform an ultrasound. The doctor will probably give you a group B streptococcus test as well, to check for an infection that about 35 percent of all adults carry, but which is usually harmless, unless it is passed on to the baby. If this happens, it can cause infections in the bloodstream, pneumonia, meningitis, or stillbirth. The risks are highest if the baby is born early or if there is a long period between the water breaking and birth.

Week 37

By the end of this week, your baby will weigh about 6.5 pounds and be about 14 inches in length from head to buttocks. This is the time for you to enjoy your pregnancy and try to relax. You may become irritated at people because it seems as if they are constantly asking when you are going to have the baby or telling you that you look like you are about to pop. It is difficult for you to remember they are well-meaning; try not to knock them out.

Your baby will continue to develop fat, and the skin will continue to lose its wrinkles. Your baby continues to imitate your breathing movements. Your cervix may begin to dilate this week as your body prepares for labor. You may also lose your mucus plug at any time between this week and week 40. Make sure you contact your doctor about any discharge you may experience.

You may find you begin to leak colostrum as you finish out your third trimester. If you do not, don't worry—there is no reason to worry that your milk won't come in when the baby needs it.

Week 38

If your baby is born this week or after, he or she is considered full-term because the baby is fully developed and can be up to about 21 inches long from head to toe. The baby should weigh around 7 pounds, and this is a good time for you to begin understanding the difference between pre-labor, labor, and false labor.

At this point, you only have, at best, a few more weeks to prepare for birth. Pack your overnight bag and the baby's diaper bag to be ready for the hospital. You also want to make sure everything at home is prepared for the baby, including a car seat for bringing the baby home.

You may find you are watching for any sign of labor, specifically for your water to break, but the fact is that only 10 percent of women's waters break on their own. Most of the time, the doctor has to break the water after they are already in labor. It is a good idea at this point to stay close to home, avoiding any long-distance trips or vacations, just in case the baby comes early.

Your baby is still growing, but at about an ounce per day, and meconium continues to accumulate in the baby's intestines. This will become the baby's first bowel movement soon after birth. The baby's head and abdomen are about the same size in circumference, and all of the sexual organs in both males and females are completely formed.

Week 39

You are almost there! Your baby is about 21 inches long and weighs about 7 pounds. The baby is fully developed, and you can go into labor at any time. You should pay attention to signs of labor, which are contractions that come in regular intervals without stopping, pink discharge, and backache.

You may find you have a lot of pressure on your bladder, causing increased urination. You may also have a hard time sleeping.

This week you should make sure that everything is prepared for you to bring your baby home.

Week 40

You have made it! You will now experience what it is like to go through labor and delivery. If you are delivering vaginally, labor starts when your cervix begins to dilate, then contractions will start at regular intervals. The next stage of labor is when you deliver the baby, and the third stage is the delivery of the placenta.

After your baby is born, the doctor will clean the mucus out of the baby's mouth and nose and cut the umbilical cord. The doctor will also carry out a series of quick screenings in order to assess your baby's vital signs. Your baby will then be measured and weighed.

After you give birth, you will experience vaginal bleeding, which can last for up to 6 weeks, breast engorgement, and postpartum depression. If you think you suffer from postpartum depression, make sure you discuss this with your doctor.

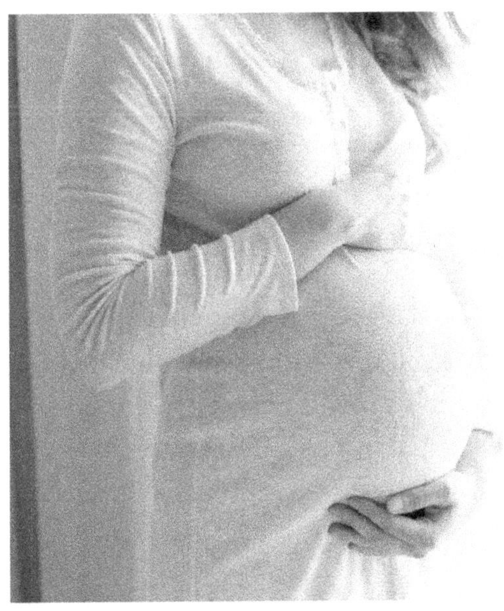

CHAPTER EIGHT

Preparing for Labor and Delivery

The 9 months of pregnancy leading up to your baby's birth provide ample time to prepare and learn everything you need to know about babies. It is also a good time to inform yourself about labor and delivery as mental preparation is a powerful thing and can help you feel more confident and controlled going into labor. From the time that those first contractions start to the final stage of active labor and delivery, there are circumstances and stages that are good to be informed about beforehand, like the early signs of labor, stages of labor, C-section, and things you need to prepare to take to the hospital.

Early Signs of Labor

Many women worry that they won't be able to recognize the signs of early labor when they occur, but luckily, the body generally knows what to do, and there is more than one sign of early labor to watch for.

Lower Back Pain
Also known as the "latent phase," early labor often begins with lower-back pain that is persistent and doesn't lessen with a change of position. Some women describe it as similar to the pain and discomfort of menstrual cramps. Often pressure applied by your partner to your lower back can help ease the pain associated with this stage.

Contractions
Sometimes early labor starts with contractions. In early labor, contractions can be painful or just feel like tightening. Most often,

they are irregular and can come and go. Early labor contractions can start right before labor begins or even arrive days or weeks before.

Breaking of the Waters

The breaking of the waters is often the tell-tale sign that labor has truly begun. It is the labor scene captured in movies that we are most familiar with. It is, however, often not as dramatic as the movies make it out to be. The membranes can rupture in a gush or a trickle. The breaking of the waters is a sign that the body is readying and approaching labor and delivery. Whether or not you leave for the hospital at this time, you should alert your health care provider that your waters have broken, and they will likely advise you to come to the hospital.

Bloody Show

Another common sign that labor begins is known as "bloody show." This is the passing of the mucus plug that blocks and protects the cervix. Once the mucus plug is passed, it could mean that labor is about to start immediately, or it could be as far as a few days away; every woman is different. Many women feel a feeling of pressure release and pass their mucus plug in the toilet with a contraction or urination.

Tummy Troubles

Women often report having an upset tummy prior to labor starting. Often, loose bowels accompany the upset tummy as the body is softening and preparing for labor.

Stages of Labor

While the duration and intensity of labor differ from woman to woman, there are designated stages of labor: early, active, and transition.

Early Labor

During the early labor stage, your body begins preparing for the upcoming delivery. Back pain, bloody show, and contractions can mark this stage. Generally, this is the longest stage of labor, and contractions can come and go and vary in intensity, but they typically get stronger as time goes on. Early labor is known to last anywhere from 8 to 12 hours. Generally, your cervix will dilate to 3 cms during this stage.

Active Labor

The active labor phase is generally when you will want to head to the hospital. Your contractions will become more painful, frequent, and regular. This is the time to put all those relaxation techniques and breathing exercises you learned in Lamas class to good use. This is also a good time to use the shower or bath to help lessen and manage the pain. Position changes are also very effective during this stage. Most often, the active phase of labor will dilate your cervix from 3 cms to 7 cms.

Transition Phase

The transition phase is where things can progress quite quickly. It is usually the shortest stage but can last anywhere from 30 minutes to 2 hours. Contractions will come very close together, and it is during this phase that your cervix completes its full dilation in preparation for the delivery. This is when the pushing will start after full dilation has occurred. During the transition phase, the cervix will complete its dilation journey and end at 10 cms. The transitional phase will end with the delivery of your baby and the passing of the placenta. Generally, a few extra pushes after delivery is enough to deliver the placenta.

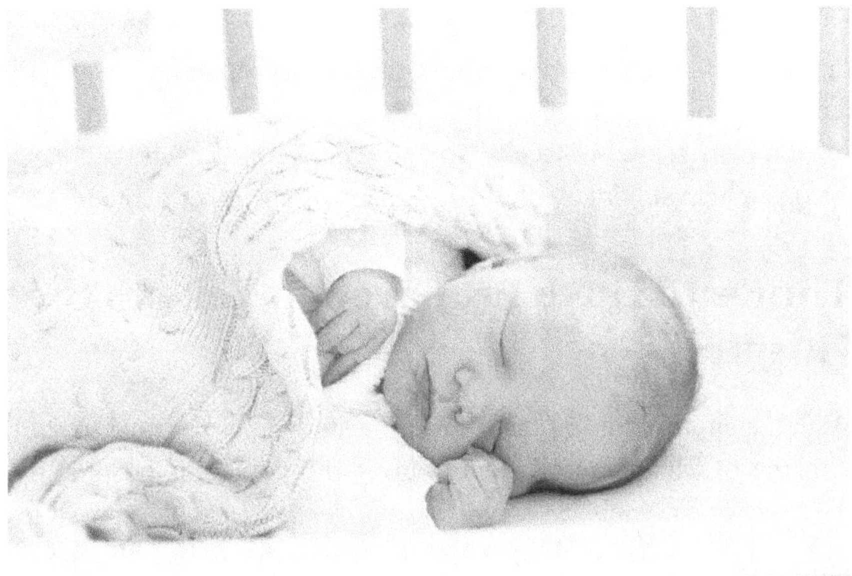

C-section

While many women, especially in their first pregnancy, approach labor and delivery with a firm idea of what they want their experience to be, sometimes the body or baby does not cooperate. If a vaginal delivery is not possible, often, a C-section is the delivery method of choice.

Otherwise known as "cesarean section," a C-section occurs when an incision is made in the mother's abdomen and uterus through which the baby is delivered. The surgical incision is made, and the baby is lifted out through the hole made by the incision.

In the event that unforeseen circumstances arise during labor where the mother or baby is in danger, or when the labor is going in too long, and the mother cannot cope, an emergency C-section may be performed. Approximately 32 percent of American women gave birth via C-sections in 2015.

Recovery from a C-section, whether planned or emergency, differs from recovery after vaginal deliveries. Your stay in the hospital will likely be longer and can last 2 to 4 days. Your surgical incision will be monitored for any signs of infection, and you will have to avoid any heavy lifting. Post-labor recovery from a C-section is measured in weeks, so you will need to ensure you have adequate help at home with the new baby or any other demands.

Things to Have Prepared to Take to the Hospital

With the approaching of that third trimester comes the time to start thinking of what you will want to take with you to the hospital. In the event of early labor, you will want to be as prepared as possible, so having your overnight bag and the baby's diaper bag all packed and ready to go is a good measure.

Infant Car Seat

First of all, you will want to have everything you need to bring the baby home safely. You and your baby will not be allowed to leave unless you have a safe car seat appropriate for newborns. A nurse will likely check that the baby is secured in the car seat safely and properly before you will be allowed to leave the hospital.

Diapers and Clothes

Other items you will need for the baby immediately are diapers and clothes. You will need newborn diapers, and if there is a special outfit you want your baby coming home in, be sure that it is clean, packed, and ready to go. People choosing to give their baby a pacifier will want to bring that, as well as some swaddling clothes and receiving blankets.

Infant Formula

If you know you will not be able to breastfeed or choose not to, you will want to bring formula and bottles so you will be able to feed your baby. If you are planning to breastfeed, a nursing bra and a breastfeeding pillow can come in handy.

Things for Mom

When you go into the hospital for labor and delivery, there is no way to know exactly how long you will be there, so it is best to prepare for a more extended stay to ensure you have everything you could need. Slippers, a bathrobe, some lotion, lip balm, any other comforts of home you think you will need should be packed.

A change of clothes or two is a must, as well as a list of phone numbers of people you will want to notify when the baby is born. A camera is also a necessity that should be pre-packed to ensure all those magical moments are captured. If you have any dietary restrictions or requirements, a snack bag is a good idea as hospital food might not suffice.

Labor and delivery is a different experience for all women. Some experience long labors and some short. Some report high pain levels, while some find that the labor is not as painful as expected. From the early stages of labor to active, transitional, and delivery, your body will surprise you with what it can do and how instinctual it can be. Some women find that while they were fully prepared for the labor and delivery stage, they are unprepared for the recovery stage. Whether you deliver vaginally or by a C-section, you will need to be prepared for adequate recovery time and make sure that you have the help you will need.

CHAPTER NINE

Postpartum: The First Days

Your body has undergone one of its most remarkable experiences, which involved growing another human being. After 9 months of anticipation, you are excited to finally have your new baby in your arms. Much of your energy and concentration during the upcoming weeks and months will be on the new addition. However, it is also important to take care of yourself.

You might have had an easy or complicated delivery. You might have had a vaginal delivery or a C-section. You might have labored for a few days or a few hours. Regardless of how it went down, your body has endured trauma and will need time to recover. Below are some guidelines and general information on how to recover from childbirth:

Newborn Care

If you have spent little or no time around newborns, you might be intimidated by their fragility. A few newborn care basics are outlined below:

• Wash your hands thoroughly or use hand sanitizer before handling your newborn. At this stage, he or she will have a weak immune system and will be at risk for infection. Ensure that everyone holding or touching your baby has clean hands.

• His or her head and neck must always be supported. When carrying the baby, cradle the head, and when carrying him or her upright or laying your baby down, ensure the head is supported.

• Your newborn should never be shaken, whether out of frustration or while playing. Shaking could result in brain bleeding or even death. When waking your infant, instead of shaking, gently blow on a cheek or tickle his or her.

• Ensure your baby is fastened securely into the car seat, stroller, or carrier. Limit activities that could be excessively bouncy or rough.

• Newborns are not ready for rough play like being thrown in the air or bounced on the knee.

Taking Baby Home

Whether your newborn immediately comes home from the hospital or comes later, his or her homecoming is a major event you have possibly often imagined. Below are tips on how to be prepared:

Leaving the Hospital
Typically, expectant moms pack outfits for the ride home before getting to the hospital. However, there are others who wait to determine what the weather will be like and have someone bring appropriate clothing. Plan on bringing loose-fitting clothing for yourself with an elastic or drawstring waist to maximize comfort.

Often, babies are overdressed for the ride home. Ensure your baby is dressed as how you would dress yourself. Therefore, if you would be hot in a knitted hat in the summer, so would your baby.

Dress your baby in light cotton pants and a T-shirt, or put a blanket over his or her bare legs. If it is cold, put on a hat, footie pajamas, and warm blanket over him or her. To avoid suffocation, ensure the blanket is far from the face.

Your baby is more likely to be calm and contented if a lot of time is not spent at the hospital attempting to dress him or her in an intricate outfit that requires pulling and pushing of limbs.

Be sure to ask when the baby's first checkup should be scheduled prior to leaving the hospital. Some premature babies leave the hospital with a special monitor to check heart rate and breathing. You might be instructed on how to administer infant cardiopulmonary resuscitation (CPR).

Whether full-term or premature, do not feel rushed out the hospital door; ensure your questions are all answered before leaving.

Car Ride

A proper child safety seat is the most essential item for the ride home. It is required by every state for parents to have one before leaving the hospital. This is because it is among the best methods of protecting your newborn.

Even on a short trip, holding your baby in your arms is dangerous. A quick stop could see your baby being pulled from your arms and hurled against the dashboard.

Before your baby is born, consider renting, buying, or borrowing a car seat. When it comes to babies, there are two types of car seats: infant-only seats and convertible seats. Infant-only seats must be switched when the baby weighs between 22 and 35 pounds. Convertible seats are designed to accommodate infants and older babies.

In addition, infant-only seats are intended solely for rear-facing use and better accommodate infants compared to convertible seats. The American Academy of Pediatrics recommends that babies travel in a rear-facing seat until they reach the maximum height and weight limits proposed by the manufacturer or until they are 2 years old. If your child surpasses the recommended weight and height before his or her second birthday, a convertible seat will be needed, which is designed for larger babies.

Some parents find that a "travel system" that comprises a stroller and an infant-only car seat, which can be affixed to the stroller, makes for a much smoother transition. This is particularly true when moving sleeping babies from the car to the stroller.

The convertible seats should be rear-facing until the baby reaches the maximum height and weight limits advised by the manufacturer or until the baby is at least 2 years of age. For a baby who gets to the weight and height limits before age 2, a bigger convertible seat that is rear-facing is the safest. Smaller kids can stay in rear-facing seats beyond age 2. Be guided by the manufacturer's recommendations for the right time to turn the car seat.

A convertible or rear-facing infant seat should never be placed in the front seat of the car. Passenger-side airbags are unsafe for both types of car seats, and most crashes impact the front passenger section of the vehicle. During the cold months, snugly strap in your baby and then place blankets over him or her.

If you opt to borrow a car seat, ensure it has never been in a crash and is not more than 6 years old. Even if a car seat that was involved in a crash looks fine, it could be unsound structurally. Avoid seats that are missing parts or do not have the manufacturer's model number and date; there will be no way of knowing about recalls.

Postpartum Recovery for Mom

Your postpartum recovery will take a while. Completely recovering from pregnancy and childbirth could actually take months. Many women feel largely recovered by 6 to 8 weeks; however, it could take longer to feel like yourself. During this period, you might feel as if your body is fighting against you but try not to become frustrated. The best things to do for your body are eat well, rest, and give yourself a break.

Additionally, your hormones will be fluctuating during this period. You will be more emotional, and thinking clearly may become challenging. Allow yourself time for these feelings to pass. However, if at any point you consider hurting your baby or yourself, talk to someone about it.

Bear in mind that each new mom is different; therefore, each woman will recover at her own rate and experience distinct postpartum symptoms. Most of the symptoms get less intense within a week. However, backaches, sore nipples, perineal pain, and other symptoms may continue for weeks. Still, others, such as leaky breasts and backache, could last until your baby is a bit older.

If you experienced a vaginal birth, perhaps you are wondering when the soreness will disappear and your perineum will heal. Recovery could take between 3 weeks if no tearing happened and more than 6 weeks if you had an episiotomy or perineal tear.

If your baby was delivered via C-section, anticipate spending between 3 and 4 days in the hospital recovering. It typically takes between 4 and 6 weeks before you feel like you are back to normal.

Breastfeeding Basics

Whether your newborn is being fed by breast or a bottle, you might be confused about how frequently to do so. Typically, it is recommended that the baby is fed on demand whenever he or she seems hungry. Your baby could cry as a cue, suck his or her finger, or make sucking noises.

Newborn babies need to be fed every 2 to 3 hours. If you are breastfeeding, make your baby nurse for approximately 10 to 15 minutes at both breasts. If your baby is fed formula, he or she will perhaps take approximately 2 to 3 ounces at each feeding.

You may need to wake up your newborn every few hours to ensure he or she is getting enough to eat. However, if you have to wake up your baby to feed often, or if he or she has trouble sucking or eating, call your pediatrician for advice.

If your newborn appears satisfied, produces several stools per day and roughly 6 wet diapers, is gaining weight consistently, and sleeps well, he or she is most likely eating enough.

Another way of telling whether your baby is getting any milk is to take note if your breasts feel full before feeding and emptier after feeding. Consult with your doctor if there are any concerns about the feeding schedule or growth of your baby.

Babies tend to swallow air while feeding, which could make them fussy. To alleviate this, burp the baby frequently. Burp your newborn every 2 to 3 ounces while bottle feeding, and each time you change breasts while breastfeeding.

If your baby has gastroesophageal reflux, tends to be gassy, or appears fussy during feedings, attempt to burp him or her every 5 minutes while breastfeeding and after each ounce, while bottle-feeding.

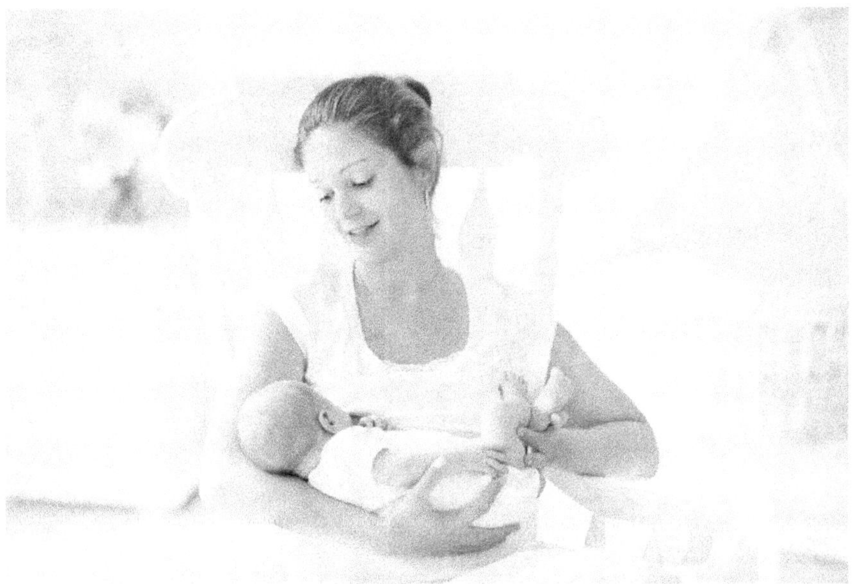

Burping Tips

• Putting his or her head on your shoulder, hold the baby in an upright position. Support the baby's back and head while using your other hand to gently pat his or her back.

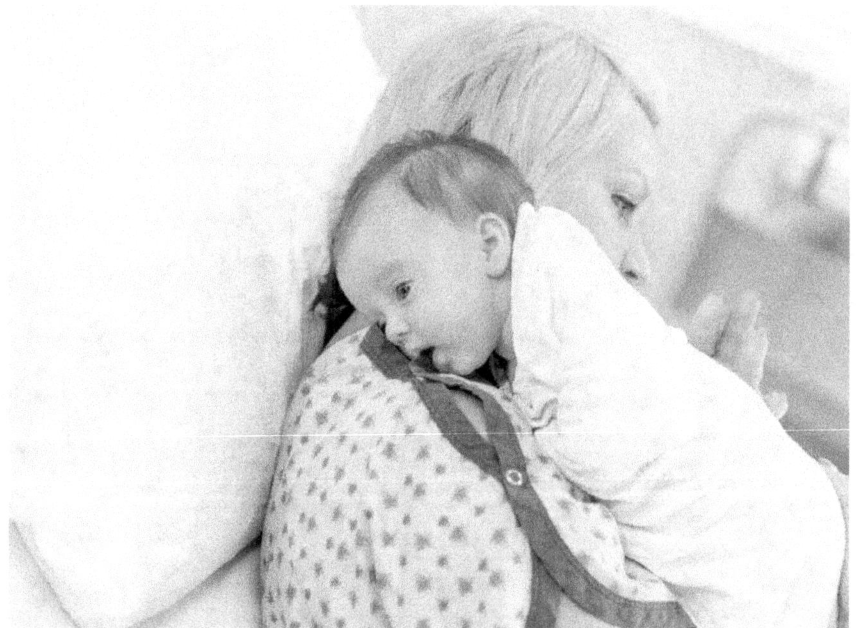

• Put the baby on your lap to sit. Use one hand to support his or her head and chest, cradling the chin in with your palm, then put the heel of your hand on his or her chest. Ensure you are gripping the baby's chin and not the throat. Gently pat the baby's back with the other hand.

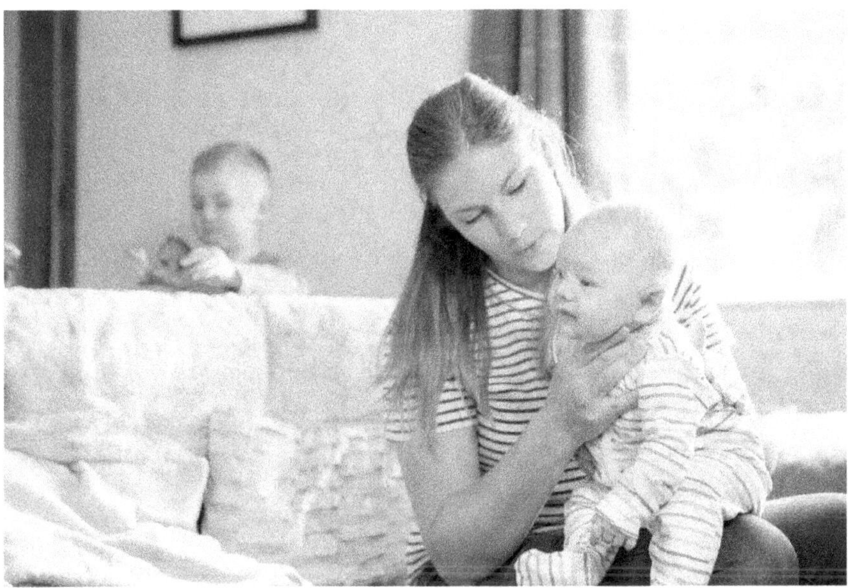

• On your lap, place the baby face-down, ensuring his or her head is supported. Ensure the head is higher than the chest while gently rubbing or patting the back.

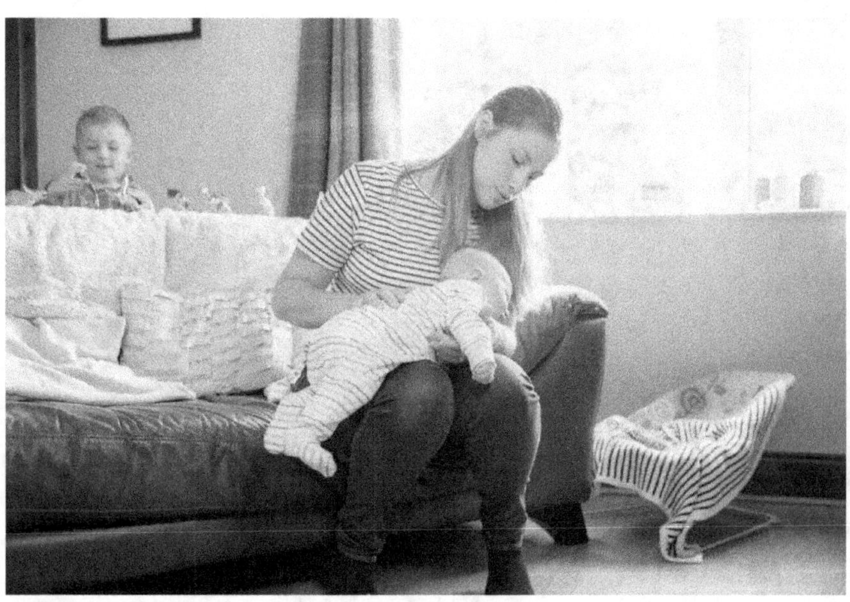

• If the baby fails to burp after a few minutes, adjust his or her position and attempt to burp for a few more minutes before feeding again. Your baby should always be burped when feeding time is over. To avoid spit-ups, keep him or her upright for a minimum of 10 to 15 minutes.

Conclusion

Pregnancy can be a scary and confusing time, but it does not have to be. By learning as much as you can about what your body will go through and how your baby is growing inside you, instead of this being a scary time, pregnancy can be beautiful. The most wonderful part of pregnancy, however, is the moment that it ends and you hold your adorable, healthy baby in your arms.

Finally, I want to thank you for reading my book. If you enjoyed the book, please share your thoughts and post a review on the book retailer's website. It would be greatly appreciated!

Best wishes,

Kimberly Ward

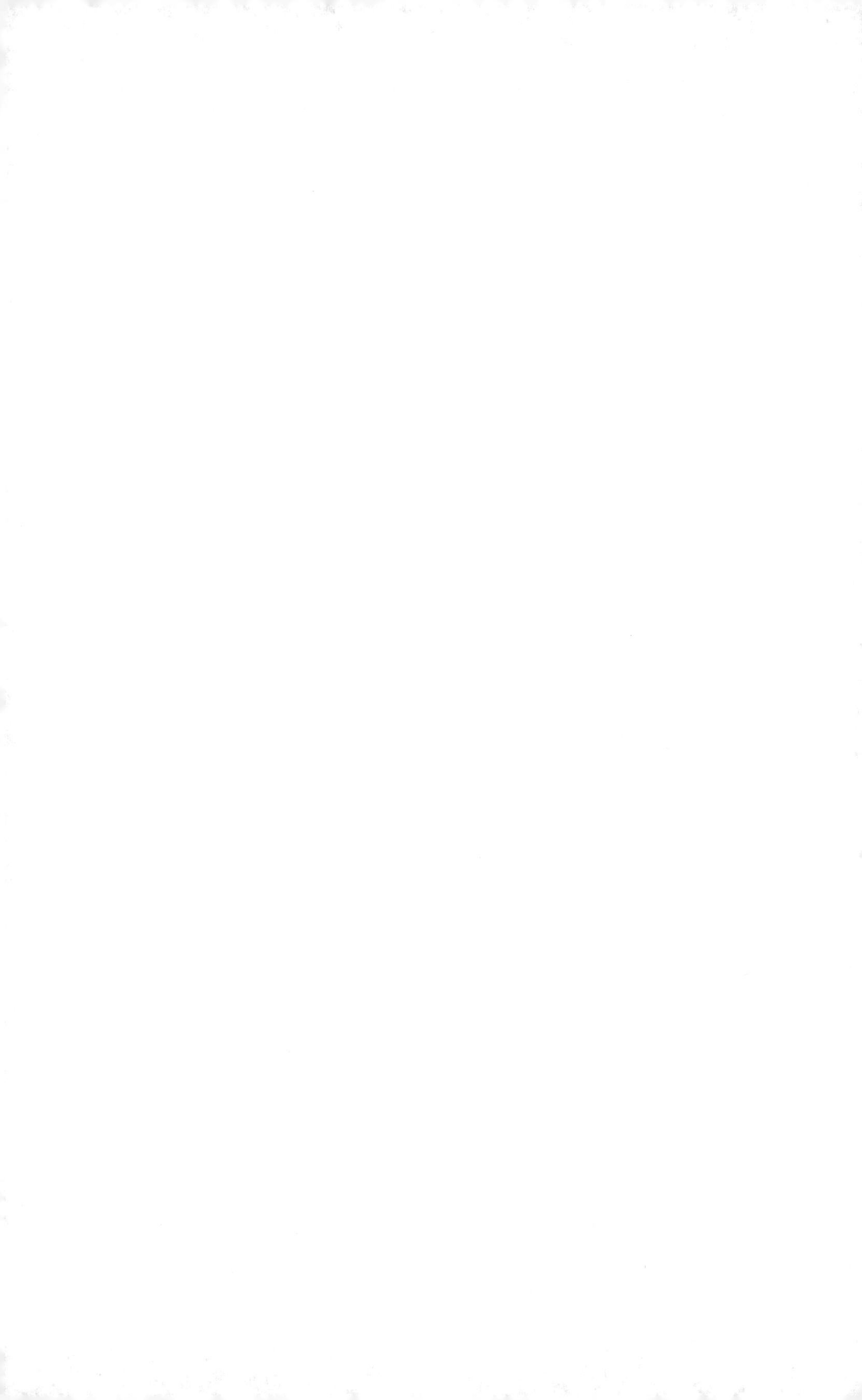